Caring for People with Learning Disabilities

A guide for non-specialist nurses

HEALTH AND SOCIAL CARE TITLES
AVAILABLE FROM LANTERN PUBLISHING LTD

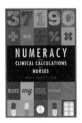
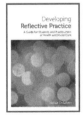
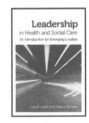
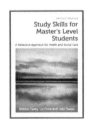
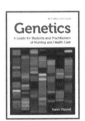

Caring for People with Learning Disabilities

A guide for non-specialist nurses

Chris Barber

Lantern

ISBN: 978 1 908625 28 1

Published in 2015 by Lantern Publishing Limited

Lantern Publishing Limited, The Old Hayloft, Vantage Business Park, Bloxham Rd, Banbury, OX16 9UX, UK

www.lanternpublishing.com

British Library Cataloguing in Publication Data

A catalogue record for this book is available from the British Library

The authors and publisher have made every attempt to ensure the content of this book is up to date and accurate. However, healthcare knowledge and information is changing all the time so the reader is advised to double-check any information in this text on drug usage, treatment procedures, the use of equipment, etc. to confirm that it complies with the latest safety recommendations, standards of practice and legislation, as well as local Trust policies and procedures. Students are advised to check with their tutor and/or mentor before carrying out any of the procedures in this textbook.

Typeset by Medlar Publishing Solutions Pvt Ltd, India

Cover design by Andrew Magee Design Ltd

Printed in the UK

Distributed by NBN International, 10 Thornbury Rd, Plymouth, PL6 7PP, UK

CONTENTS

ABOUT THE AUTHOR

The author is a registered nurse (learning disabilities), qualifying as such in December 1989. He has worked in a wide variety of clinical settings, both residential and community, with a wide variety of service users (those who are on the autism spectrum, those with sensory impairments, those whose behaviour 'challenges services', those who require forensic services and care and those with mental health issues). He is a parent of a young man who is also on the autism spectrum and he himself was diagnosed at the end of 2008 as being 'high-functioning autistic'. He holds an MEd from the University of Birmingham in special educational needs (autism). He sits on the editorial board of the *British Journal of Nursing* and the *British Journal of Health Care Assistants,* and as well as having written a number of articles/papers on a wide variety of subjects including learning disabilities, care givers, spirituality and autism, he is the author of *Autism and Asperger's Conditions,* published by Quay Books.

FOREWORD

This is a beautifully and sensitively written book. Although it has been aimed at health care professionals and students, it is equally applicable to carers and families of people living with learning disabilities. It follows the life course of those with learning disabilities, and the use of case studies makes it an exceptionally realistic information guide. Every chapter is significant and has a crucial role in the care and nurturing of this population.

Three of the themes covered touched me in particular. Firstly, at a time when dementia care is at the forefront of delivery of appropriate care and support, it is encouraging to highlight the condition and its impact on people with learning disability as overall life expectancy increases. Using the scenarios to support the level of care, and addressing the gaps in care provision for people with learning disability, assists in increasing awareness for health workers.

In *Chapter 9*, the author covers a subject that health care professionals, families and carers alike find it difficult to mention and even discuss with the person with the learning disability. It is, in my view, important that sexuality is not treated as a taboo subject but as a human right, with the appropriate support to change attitudes of stakeholders and carers.

In *Chapter 12*, informal carers are addressed; these are unpaid carers whose needs and wellbeing are often ignored or overlooked. The author examines this and offers the reader an understanding of the important role they play and the need to be rewarded for their contribution. Thank you to you all.

Chris Barber's book is an enjoyable, touching and inspirational read for all those involved in the lives of people with learning disabilities.

Cecilia Anim
President of the Royal College of Nursing (2015)

ACKNOWLEDGEMENTS

I would like to thank my wife Jean and my son Freddie for their support and patience during the writing of this book.

Furthermore, I would like to thank the reviewers for their kind and thoughtful comments and suggestions regarding the text.

Finally, I would like to thank Mark Allen Publishing for their kind permission to reproduce text that was first published by the *British Journal of Health Care Assistants*.

01

INTRODUCTION

This book is intended for those health care assistants, nursing students and staff nurses who are not learning disability specialists but who, as a result of working with those who have a learning disability, would like to learn more about and understand learning disability as a condition and hence provide better care and support for those with a learning disability. As the following three boxes show, learning disability registered nurses are facing and are likely to continue to face a number of professional challenges. Consequently, the support that the non-learning disability specialist will be able to offer both those with a learning disability and learning disability nurses is likely to become increasingly important.

> "At a time when the number of people with learning difficulties is growing, the size of the learning disability workforce is shrinking, along with available nursing support"
>
> (Lowthian, 2011, page 6)

> "There are currently big issues for learning disability nurses around networks of support and a sense of isolation when it comes to accessing them. At present there's nothing in place to assist the learning disability workforce"
>
> (Michael Brown, Chair of the RCN's learning disability forum as cited by Lowthian, 2011, page 6)

> "Learning disability nurses need to be given sufficient training, status and recognition by the NHS. Without this recognition, fewer nurses will choose to specialise in this area and the quality of care offered will only get worse"
>
> (David Congdon (Mencap) as cited by Lowthian, 2011, page 6)

Indeed, given these professional challenges facing many learning disability nurses, it is possible for the non-specialist health care assistant (HCA), student nurse or staff nurse to come into their own here and make a significant and positive impact upon the care experienced by those who have a learning disability.

Why the need for another book on learning disability nursing, care and support? Indeed, is there a need?

This may seem to be a slightly odd way to open a new book which aims to support those who provide non-specialist nursing, health and social care support for those with learning disabilities, as there are a number of other books that will be useful in supporting and caring for both adults and children with learning disabilities. Mark Jukes (2009), Ian Peate and Debra Fearns (2006), Louise Clark and Peter Griffiths (2008) and Helena Priest and Michael Gibbs (2011) spring to mind here. There are also an increasing number of books about autism spectrum conditions that may be of use, including Barber (2011). However, the reason for this book is to provide the non-learning disability specialist care professional with practical suggestions, which are easy to both follow and implement, for supporting this client group. It is not the intention to replicate the contents of other books but to highlight areas that seem to 'fall between the cracks' and consequently are rarely if ever mentioned within other books: discrimination, spirituality, 'informal care givers' and sexuality, as well as dying, death and bereavement. Please, do not be put off by the occasional 'confrontational' comment that may be found within these pages. It is not meant to suggest that nursing care for those with a learning disability is poor; indeed, far from it! However, there may be occasions when the attitudes and practices of some HCAs, nursing students and registered nurses may need to be challenged. If through the process of this challenging, people have been offended, then apologies are offered and forgiveness sought.

As can be seen from the quotes that began this chapter, we live and work in interesting times. There are a large number of books, journals and journal articles by countless authors around those with a learning disability, the families of those with a learning disability, learning disability nurses and learning disability care workforce in general. However, there still appears to be a real and serious gap in the knowledge of many non-specialist nurses, doctors, social care staff and the 'professions allied to medicine' (PAMS: physiotherapists, occupational therapists and paramedics) regarding the lives and needs of those with a learning disability.

Let me pose a small number of simple challenges:

PAUSE FOR THOUGHT 1.1

How much do you *really* know about learning disability and those with a learning disability?

PAUSE FOR THOUGHT 1.2

In any given week where you work, how many of your patients or service users do you think have a learning disability?

PAUSE FOR THOUGHT 1.3

Is your knowledge of learning disability enough to provide the type and level of care and support that you would like and that your patients or service users need?

If the non-learning disability specialist nurse, nursing student or health care assistant experiences challenges such as these, this may well impact upon the quality of care that those with a learning disability could experience (Mencap, 2007).

As far back as 1979, the Jay Report (Jay Committee, 1979) recommended the ending of learning disability as a nursing branch. Such recommendations have been echoed over many years during debates at RCN Congress. Even the Nursing and Midwifery Council (2008) tried to restructure pre-registration nurse training with a view to establishing a generalist nurse who would, in theory, have enough knowledge and skills to work in any clinical setting and with any clinical group. Learning disability, mental health and paediatric branches could all be followed at post-registration level. Indeed, such an approach received much, but by no means universal support within nursing's senior management and senior leadership, and was also resisted by many nurses. It may be likely that groups of other health care workers such as physiotherapists, occupational therapists and paramedics may also be debating their roles in engaging with and supporting those with a learning disability whom they encounter through their work.

But what of the roles of the 'non-learning disability' nurse, nursing student, HCA, physiotherapist, occupational therapist, paramedic or social care worker? After all, one criticism that could be levelled, possibly with some validity, at existing books is that perhaps the bulk of these books that are available on the subject of learning disability and the care and support of those with a learning disability are aimed, primarily, at those working within the field of learning disability care and support. However, do not all nurses, HCAs, social care staff and many physiotherapists, occupational therapists and paramedics come into contact and work with people with a learning disability at some point in their careers?

Partly to answer this criticism, four 'colleagues' would like to introduce themselves:

Sally is a senior staff nurse with five years' post-qualifying experience, first in an A&E department and then in an acute medical ward of her local general hospital. Sally says that she occasionally encounters patients who have a learning disability but does not feel confident in meeting their specific care needs.

Hanif is a '40-something' second-year student nurse who is following the 'adult branch'. Before commencing his nurse training, Hanif worked as an HCA in the same A&E department as Sally. Hanif would like to learn more about learning disability than he feels that he currently learns from his training.

Jill is an HCA who has worked at her local GP practice and community health centre for the past six years after working in an office for a year. Jill has a younger sister who has Down's syndrome.

Chris is a registered nurse for those with a learning disability and is the author of this, his second book. Chris, who has Asperger's syndrome/high-functioning autism, currently works as a full-time care giver for his wife and son.

Sally, Hanif and Jill have very kindly asked to act as 'critical and questioning friends' who will ask the odd question and make the occasional comment and observation on the care and support of those with a learning disability from their own perspectives and experiences. Chris will re-appear in the final chapter.

A BRIEF OVERVIEW OF THE BOOK

In order to fill some of these gaps in knowledge and understanding, this short book will focus on a number of issues pertinent to the understanding, care and support of those with a learning disability.

At this point, Marcel, Ziva and Thomas would like to introduce themselves.

Marcel is a '30-something' man who was born in Morocco and who happens to have Down's syndrome. He lives at home with his parents who are in their 60s and his pet cat that he calls 'Moggy'. Marcel works part time at the café at his local supermarket. His elder sister, Ziva, is married and has two children. Marcel's hobbies include music, 'Red Dwarf', country walks and meeting people.

Ziva, who is Marcel's sister, has Asperger's syndrome/high-functioning autism. She is married and has two children, one of whom is also on the autism spectrum. Ziva works part time as a university lecturer in pure and applied maths.

Thomas is 65 years old and has a profound and multiple learning disability with additional severe mobility problems, pre-verbal communication skills, inability to digest food, arthritis and epilepsy. Thomas lives within a social care home.

Marcel, Ziva and Thomas have asked if they can be your guides throughout the following chapters.

Chapter 2 gives a definition of learning disability. There are a number of definitions and unless one is able to understand what learning disability is, it could be suggested that health and social care and support of those with a learning disability will be impoverished. The lived meaning and experience of having a learning disability will be highlighted through the eyes of Marcel, Ziva and Thomas.

The meaning of profound and multiple learning disability will be focused on in *Chapter 3* and will be informed by the experiences of Thomas.

There have been many government and independent sector reports over the last 40 years or so around the services for, and the quality of life of those with a learning disability. These have included reports into some of the learning disability hospitals in the early 1970s, the Jay Report in the late 1970s, the 2001 White Paper (*'Valuing People'*) and the Mencap report *'Death by Indifference'* in 2007. *Chapter 4* will focus on and explain what these reports and any subsequent legislation mean for nurses, nursing students, HCAs, social care staff and PAMs working with people with a learning disability.

Many, if not most nurses and HCAs are likely, at some point in their work, to encounter and provide health care support to those with a learning disability. *Chapter 5* will focus on how to provide high quality support within a number of generalist health care environments including health centres, GP practices, outpatient departments and acute/medical or surgical wards of a general hospital.

Chapter 6 will focus on the often complex area of consent to treatment and intervention with regards to those with a learning disability. Just because a person has a learning disability does not necessarily mean that they cannot give, withhold or withdraw consent.

Although learning disability and mental ill health **are not** the same thing, there is an overlap between the two. *Chapter 7* will focus on the mental health needs of those with a learning disability.

Some of those with a learning disability will commit crimes; occasionally, some of these crimes will be of a very serious nature including assault, murder, sexual assault, rape and arson and will require specialist forensic services. *Chapter 8* will focus on the care and support of those with a learning disability who require such specialist services.

The subject of sexuality, relationships and those with a learning disability as parents has always been very controversial. *Chapter 9* will focus on the sexual and relationship needs of those with a learning disability.

The challenges and delights of ageing for those with a learning disability and those who care for them will be highlighted in *Chapter 10*.

Although learning disability does not necessarily equate to having a short life span as once it did, dying and death are part and parcel and are the inevitable conclusion of all life, of all humanity. *Chapter 11* will focus on end of life processes and the role of the nurse and HCA in this process.

Many, if not most, people with a learning disability will live at home with their parents and siblings rather than in a non-family residential setting such as a learning disability hospital or community home. *Chapter 12* will focus on the experiences and needs of families who look after a person with a learning disability.

There has been a long and very sad and painful history of discrimination against those with a learning disability and their families. Following on from the previous chapter on the care and support of 'informal carers', *Chapter 13* will focus on this history and the role of the nurse, HCA, social care staff and PAMs in combating such discrimination and prejudice.

Spirituality is not about ticking the 'Church of England' box on the service user's assessment form or attention to the cultural and religious dimensions of diet, clothing and personal hygiene. *Chapter 14* will focus on and explore a definition and applicability of spirituality to those with a learning disability.

The final chapter will look back and reflect in order to look forward, with a view to suggesting a small number of future developments in learning disability services and care. This chapter will also include a conversation between Hanif, Ziva, Thomas, Sally, Marcel and Jill.

The appendices comprise a brief glossary of learning disability terms and a short selection of resources on learning disability, those with a learning disability and practical suggestions on how to support those with a learning disability.

Ziva, being a university lecturer, may be an odd person to act as a guide in a book about learning disabilities as the inclusion of Asperger's syndrome, or high-functioning autism as it is sometimes known, in the umbrella term of learning disability is debatable. However, Ziva says that she will delve into this issue in the next chapter. On the other hand, being Marcel's sister, she is able to provide much useful information regarding life with a learning disability. The stories of Thomas, Marcel and Ziva will unfold over the coming pages and chapters, but at the moment they would just like to say "Hi"!

All that remains to be said here is welcome to this short book. I hope that you will enjoy reading it, that it will challenge how you think about and interact with those who have a learning disability and that it will be of use and benefit to you in your daily work.

REFERENCES

Barber, C. (2011) *Autism and Asperger's Conditions: a practical guide for nurses.* London, Quay Books.

Clark, L. & Griffiths, P. (2008) *Learning Disability and Other Intellectual Impairments.* Chichester, John Wiley.

Department of Health (2001) *Valuing People: a new strategy for learning disabilities for the 21st century.* London, HMSO.

Jay Committee (1979) *The Report of the Committee of Enquiry into Mental Handicap Nursing and Care.* London, Department of Health/HMSO.

Jukes, M. (2009) *Learning Disability Nursing Practice.* London, Quay Books.

Lowthian, S. (2011) *Strengthening the Learning Disability Workforce.* RCN Bulletin.

Mencap (2007) *Death by Indifference.* London, Mencap. Available at: www.mencap.org.uk/sites/default/files/documents/2008-03/DBIreport.pdf (last accessed 17 November 2014)

Nursing and Midwifery Council (2008) *The Future of Pre-registration Nurse Education.* London, NMC.

Peate, I. & Fearns, D. (2006) *Caring for People with Learning Disabilities.* Chichester, John Wiley.

Priest, H. & Gibbs, M. (2011) *Mental Health Care for People with Learning Disabilities.* Elsevier.

02

WHAT IS LEARNING DISABILITY?

AIMS AND LEARNING OUTCOMES:

The aims of this chapter are to:

- Present two 'dictionary' type definitions of 'learning disability'
- Discuss these two definitions
- Highlight the identity of learning disability.

By the end of this chapter you will have gained:

- A basic understanding of the definition and meaning of learning disability from a number of different standpoints
- A basic understanding of how these meanings have changed over time.

Marcel, a 39-year-old man with Down's syndrome is admitted, having had a stroke, onto the general medical ward on which Hanif works as part of a 2nd year student nurse placement. This is the first time that Hanif has had a patient with Down's syndrome and he knows very little about learning disability in general and Down's syndrome in particular. At the handover at the start of Hanif's shift, he asks: 'What is learning disability?'

PAUSE FOR THOUGHT 2.1

A nurse, who during a debate at RCN Congress said that he considers himself to have Asperger's syndrome, was asked: 'What is this disease called Asperger's?' Do you, the reader, consider learning disability to be a disease? Do you consider that learning disability is catching?

INTRODUCTION

What is learning disability? Hanif would be forgiven for asking this question, particularly as he has not previously worked with people who have a learning disability. Following on from this initial question, it may be appropriate that a number of further questions could be asked: What does it mean to *have* a learning disability? Indeed, to develop this further, what does it mean to *be* 'learning disabled'?

A careful reading of the above questions seems to highlight three different issues:

- A possible need for a basic, clear and factual definition of learning disability
- A possible need for a discussion around learning disability as *possession* in much the same way as having or possessing a broken leg or a broken arm or having a headache
- A possible need for a discussion around learning disability as personal identity.

These are all valid and perfectly reasonable questions to ask, particularly if Hanif has had very little if any previous knowledge or experience of, or exposure to learning disability as either an 'abstract' or a 'physical' concept or reality. Appropriate theoretical learning and clinical experience opportunities around learning disabilities may not always be available to Hanif.

Again, there could well be a perception that learning disability is a 'childhood' condition or there may well be some confusion as to 'learning disabilities' and 'learning difficulties', with some people thinking that these two terms refer to the same condition or phenomenon. *Learning difficulties* or *specific learning difficulties* usually refer to the specific conditions of dyslexia, dyspraxia and dyscalculia. Specific Learning Difficulties (SpLDs) affect the way information is learned and processed. They are neurological (rather than psychological), usually run in families and occur independently of intelligence. They can have significant impact on education and learning and on the acquisition of literacy skills (British Dyslexia Association, 2012).

Hanif, as both a pre-registration nursing student and a future post-registration staff nurse, is very likely to encounter and work with those who have a learning disability in his day-to-day work, regardless of whether he works in a general hospital, in the community or in a GP practice or health centre. As such, Marcel's sister, Ziva, would like to act as Hanif's guide in the following pages.

DEFINITION

Hanif: So, Ziva, what does this term *'learning disability'* actually mean?

Ziva: Thanks for asking, Hanif. Barber (2011) suggested that the term 'learning disability' cannot be defined easily. Learning disability can act as a category for a variety of conditions with different causes. Some forms of learning disability are:

- As a result of 'genetic abnormalities'. Down's syndrome, phenylketonuria, Marfan's syndrome and tuberous sclerosis (epiloia) are all examples of genetic causes

- As a result of major difficulties during or immediately after childbirth
- As a result of alcohol or 'recreational drug' use during pregnancy
- As a result of environmental factors such as environmental or industrial toxins

Whilst other forms of learning disability just are (otherwise known as 'idiopathic')! An idiopathic (from the Greek *idios* ('one's own') and *pathos* ('suffering')) disease or condition is one whose cause is not known or one that arises spontaneously.

Hanif: Thanks for that, Ziva. However, what you have just presented is some of the causes of learning disability, rather than what learning disability actually is (and is not).

Ziva: Yes, you are quite right about that, Hanif. Sorry. There are a number of ways of looking at the term 'learning disability' and hence those with a learning disability. The first of these is to focus on learning disability as a 'dictionary definition'. Again, there are a number of such definitions that can be looked at. The first of these definitions is taken from the *Valuing People* White Paper (DH, 2001: 14). According to *Valuing People*, a person is described as having a learning disability if they have:

- A significantly reduced ability to understand new or complex information (impaired intelligence and cognitive functioning)

- A significantly reduced ability to learn new skills (impaired intelligence and cognitive functioning), with

- A reduced ability to cope independently (impaired social functioning) and

- Which started before adulthood and with a lasting effect on development.

Alternatively, learning disability can be seen as:

- An arrested or incomplete development of mind (Mental Health Act 1983, Section 1)

- That impacts upon most if not all areas of human life: intellectual, spiritual, physical, educational and social

- And ranges in severity and impact from borderline to profound

- With the likelihood of multiple neurological and physical disabilities increasing with serious and profound learning disabilities

- And that often requires additional supportive resources in order to facilitate optimum physical, mental, spiritual, social and emotional health and engagement within society.

Hanif: I think I understand these two meanings, Ziva.

Ziva: However, both of these definitions could be argued to pose a number of questions or problems. First: the Department of Health definition. '*Valuing People*' was the first learning disability White Paper for nearly a quarter of a century.

Hanif: What is a White Paper, Ziva?

Ziva: A White Paper is formal Government policy on a given subject such as learning disability, as opposed to a Green Paper which is a discussion or consultation document and a Bill or Act of Parliament. A White Paper has no force of law behind it and cannot, therefore, be enforced in the same way as an Act of Parliament such as the Autism Act 2009. The definition given in the White Paper is apparently the 'definition of choice' and can be found as such in many learning disability textbooks and is both concise and accurate. However, it lacks in its apparent objectivity and simplicity the possibility that learning disability is not a single condition, but a series of conditions. These conditions range from 'Borderline' learning disability through to 'Profound' learning disabilities via 'Mild', 'Moderate' and 'Severe' learning disabilities.

Hanif: Would I be right in thinking that the more severe the learning disability is, the more likely that such learning disability will include increasing physical disabilities such as cerebral palsy, musculoskeletal issues such as scoliosis, neurological conditions such as epilepsy and medical conditions such as respiratory and cardiac problems?

Ziva: Yes, you would. Again, although succinct and relatively easy to understand, it could be argued that this definition runs the risk of locating the disability within rather than outside the person. My brother Marcel is disabled and must learn to adapt to society, rather than Marcel having a disability imposed by societal attitudes and practices – attitudes and practices which prevent Marcel from fully engaging with society.

Hanif: OK. But where would one place those with Asperger's syndrome or high-functioning autism in this learning disability range?

Ziva: Interesting question, Hanif. I must declare a personal interest here as I am Asperger's. Few people would argue that 'classic autism' is not a form of learning disability, as it shares many of the cognitive issues and impairments of learning disability. However, do people such as Bill Gates (founder of Microsoft), Keith Joseph (British politician), Ludwig Wittgenstein (Austrian philosopher), Peter Sellers (British comedian) and Gary Numan (British electronic musician), all of whom are suggested to have Asperger's syndrome, fit comfortably within a traditional learning disability framework? Probably not!

Hanif: Since those with Asperger's tend to have higher than average IQs, given the names mentioned above (some of whom I know of), is Asperger's an aspect of learning disability?

Ziva: Another interesting question and the jury is still out on this one! Anyway, the second definition is based on the opening section of the 1983 Mental Health Act and probably comes closest to providing a 'legal definition' of learning disability. However, this definition also applies to those with mental health issues and is not specific to learning disability. Again, the concept of 'mind' is introduced but, sadly, is not defined or developed. Having said that, this definition appears to be more 'holistic' in tone and acknowledges that learning disability is a spectrum of conditions.

Hanif: I mentioned a moment ago the idea of IQ and learning disability. Could you talk me through this connection?

Ziva: Although this definition is now seen as outmoded, learning disability has been defined in terms of intelligence quotient (IQ), a scale which was used to measure intellectual or mental ability. In general, IQ levels indicated that (Newcastle University, 2011):

People with an IQ level of:	Were classified as:
75 and above	'Normal'
70 to 75	'Borderline' learning disability
60 to 70	'Mild' learning disability
50 to 60	'Moderate' learning disability
40 to 50	'Severe' learning disability
Less than 40	'Profound' learning disability

Hanif: I have heard that the general effectiveness of IQ ratings in indicating the level of a person's learning disability is contested as being arbitrary, crude and inaccurate (New Scientist, 2009), and may not therefore be the best method of indicating learning disability.

Ziva: You are right about that, Hanif. I too have often struggled with this concept of IQ. However, another way of viewing learning disability is to see learning disability as a combination of intellectual and physical or health conditions (Garvey and Vincent, 2006). A practical example of this view could be those with Down's syndrome, such as my brother Marcel, who are likely to experience difficulties in a number of different ways (Garvey and Vincent, 2006).

Hanif: OK, Ziva, I understand that. What are these different ways that you mention?

Ziva: These could include communication problems, a tendency to being overweight, problems with balance and mobility, painful joints and muscles, mental health issues, sensory issues, heart problems and respiratory problems. I know that this may appear to be a rather long list of health problems and there may be other health care issues that those with a learning disability may experience. However, it has to be said that not every person with a learning disability will experience all of these health issues. Again, caution must be applied here as many people who do not have a learning disability may also experience some or many of the health issues above, at some point in their lives.

Now here is a question: How many people in the UK do you think are affected by learning disability?

Ziva: Hanif, you would be forgiven if you either plucked a figure randomly out of the air or said that you did not have a clue. If you said the latter, you are not alone: estimates of how many people experience learning disabilities vary. For example, in 2001 the Department of Health (DH) estimated that there were *approximately* 1.4 million people (out of a population of around 49 million) with a learning disability in England, of whom 210 000 had a severe disability (DH, 2001). If there are approximately 63 million people living in the UK (Office for National Statistics, 2011), the DH figures would suggest that there are currently almost 1.8 million people with learning disabilities across the four nations that make up the UK, of whom about 265 000 have a severe or profound and multiple learning disability (PMLD). Mencap (2011) suggests that there are currently about 1.5 million people who have a learning disability within the UK; that is around 2.5% (or 1 person in every 40) of the UK population, given a current UK population of 60 million.

Hanif: Is the wording in *Pause for thought 2.2* a bit naughty? I spotted that the question asked how many people are *affected* by learning disability, not how many people *have* a learning disability. By asking how many people are affected by learning disability, the families, relatives, friends and even care professionals, each with their own expectations, needs and even agendas, must be included. Whilst there are between 1.5 and 1.8 million people in the UK with a learning disability, those affected by learning disability will be much higher.

BASIC HISTORY

Student nurses today will, when they qualify, register as 'Registered Nurse (*learning disability*)'. When I qualified as a learning disability nurse in 1989, my qualification was 'Registered Nurse (*mental handicap*)'. My tutors' and lecturers' qualification was 'Registered Nurse (*mental subnormality*)'.

Hanif: I notice that we have now moved on from understanding what learning disability means. Why is it important to look at the history of learning disability? After all, it is where we are now and where we are going that is important!

Ziva: I could not agree more, Hanif, but also I could not agree less! Unless you are aware of and understand the history of learning disability, how language has framed the definitions of learning disability and disability discourse, how such definitions and discourse and how those with a learning disability have been viewed have changed over time, then you may not be able to understand the present. If you cannot understand the present, there can be no future. To put this observation another way, those who do not have awareness and understanding of the past are condemned to repeat its mistakes! As can be seen from *Pause for thought 2.3*, the history of learning disability and those with a learning disability is bound intimately to language and its use. The lives of those with a learning disability and the ways that they have been treated by society in general, and health and social care professionals in particular, have changed for the better when the language that in part defines them has changed.

Hanif: Forgive my ignorance but is learning disability a recent condition? By that I mean how far back in history does learning disability go?

Ziva: Learning disability is not a recent condition by any means; it was likely that learning disability existed in biblical times. It may not have been inconceivable that learning disability, autism spectrum conditions and mental health conditions were considered to be examples of demon possession or a result of sin (Heuser, 2012; Romero, 2012). During the Middle Ages those with learning disabilities were either considered to be the 'village idiot' or due to their simplicity and naivety 'God's holy fools' and either exalted or reviled, feared and hated. Many of those with a learning disability, an autism spectrum condition or a mental health issue would have been considered to be, and condemned as witches due to their behaviour. Again, those with a learning disability would likely have been left on the street to either barely survive through begging, to be 'cared for' by the Church or to die. From 1850–1910 (Gilbert, 2009) a more 'formalised' approach to care began to emerge which seemed to coincide with changes in social philosophy and policy. Those with a learning disability were seen as harmless but 'sub-human'. The emphasis of service provision was on separation and segregation of those with either a learning disability or mental health issue from the rest of society. However, those with borderline or mild learning disabilities were considered fit for menial, largely rural, work.

Hanif: I am aware that the first half of the 20th century saw huge social upheaval. How did those with a learning disability fare?

Ziva: Well, it seems that the over-riding form of care was the 'colony' (Gilbert, 2009).

Hanif: Could you explain what you mean by the word 'colony'?

Ziva: A 'colony' was a large mental subnormality/mental handicap hospital, usually situated in rural areas. Hospitals such as South Ockendon in Essex would have been colonies. The predominant social philosophy at the time would have been one of social and gender separation and eugenics, the gradual elimination of the weakest.

Hanif: OK, not much change then. How did this change, and indeed, did it change in the latter half of the century?

Ziva: The early 1970s saw a number of public enquiries into the standard of care in many of these large hospitals, including South Ockendon in Essex and Ely in Cardiff (Gilbert, 2009). Largely as a result of these public enquiries, better services for those with a learning disability were designed, those with a learning disability were seen as consumers of care and in the 1990s there appeared a growth in disability rights and equality. There was also the growth of small family-sized community homes reflecting the growth in community integration.

Hanif: So that brings us nearly to the start of the 21ˢᵗ century.

Ziva: Yes. The new century sees the continued growth in social inclusion, human and civil rights, citizenship and self-advocacy (Gilbert, 2009). 'Mental handicap' becomes 'learning disability'. The old hospitals closed and care was (and is) provided in much smaller community-based homes. Many of those with a learning disability were encouraged to live semi-independently in their own homes with multi-agency support.

Hanif: I understand that there has also been some anti-discriminatory legislation during this time?

Ziva: Yes, Hanif. There was the Disability Discriminatory Act in 1995, the *'Valuing People'* White Paper in 2001 and the Equality Act in 2010. All of these had an impact upon those with a learning disability and will be discussed further in *Chapter 4*.

WHAT IT MEANS TO HAVE A LEARNING DISABILITY

PAUSE FOR THOUGHT 2.4

Marcel has Down's syndrome. Is he 'learning disabled' or does he have a 'learning disability'? To put this question another way: is Marcel disabled or does he have a disability?

Ziva: This question may not be either as simple or as rhetorical as it may at first seem. After all, in the previous section one can see how the use of language such as 'idiots', 'lunacy', 'mentally subnormal', 'mental handicap' and 'learning disability' changed over time and helped frame how those with a learning disability were viewed and treated.

PAUSE FOR THOUGHT 2.5

A sign noticed in a church: **'INVALID TOILET'**. Does this mean that this toilet is in-valid, not/non-valid? Or does it mean that those who use it are somehow in-valid, not valid?

Ziva: In one way, we can never really understand and appreciate what it really *means* to my brother Marcel to have a learning disability as such meanings are often 'value-laden', subjective and personal to every person who has a disability. After all, it is often claimed by those on the autism spectrum such as me, for example, that if you meet one person with autism then you have met one person with autism! However, many are likely to experience discrimination, hate-motivated crime, infantilising attitudes, a lack of understanding and poor care on the part of some (but by no means all) care professionals. It could be suggested that one of the reasons for such experiences is the nature of the disability model that has been used in order to engage with those with a learning disability. There have been two main theoretical models that have sought to explain disability: the bio-medical model of disability and the social model of disability.

Bio-medical model (Hallawell, 2009)

- The person with a learning disability is seen, addressed and treated as a patient

- The role of the patient is to comply with medical, nursing and social 'treatment'

- The focus is on the disability: the individual is considered to be disabled due to his or her impairment

- The person is defined by his or her disability

- The language around disability is one of negative terms, of deviance, lacking normality

- The disability prevents the person from fully engaging within society

- The person with disability has to change in order to fit into society.

Social model (Hallawell, 2009)

- Although originating in the mid-1970s, the social model came to prominence in the 1990s

- Has been described as being vaguely 'Marxist' in orientation

- Suggests that there is a difference between 'impairment' (such as sensory or physical impairment or learning disability) and 'disability'

- Looks beyond the individual impairment or disability to examine the social, political, educational and environmental causes of disability

- It is society that causes and imposes disability on the individual due to its ignorance, stereotyping and the erection of structural, physical, environmental and attitudinal barriers that prevent full engagement, inclusion and participation of the individual with a disability or impairment within society

- A positive disability identity and a pride in having a disability develops out of a greater control by those with a disability of both their own lives and the services that are provided for them

- An aspect of this greater control by those with a disability is independent living supported with assistance when needed, rather than communal and dependent living.

CONCLUSION

Hanif has been exposed to a number of different meanings and perspectives of learning disability. As a result, he has acquired a basic understanding of what learning disability is. The meaning and understanding of learning disability is very much multi-dimensional in nature; differences in meaning and hence understanding arise from light being shone on learning disability from a variety of different angles, from a variety of different perspectives. Again, the meaning and understanding of learning disability has changed over time and will continue to do so. This is normal!

KEY POINTS

- There is no single definition of 'learning disability'.

- The ways in which learning disability and its attendant health issues can affect a person are manifold.

- It is important to know a basic history of learning disability before the current situation can be understood and to prevent historical mistakes being repeated.

- There are different theoretical models of care, the main ones being 'social' and 'bio-medical'.

REFERENCES

Barber, C. (2011) Understanding learning disabilities: an introduction. *British Journal of Health Care Assistants*, 05:04; 169–170.

British Dyslexia Association (2012) *What are Specific Learning Difficulties?* Available at: www.bdadyslexia.org.uk/about-dyslexia/schools-colleges-and-universities/what-are-specific-learning-difficulties.html (last accessed 16 October 2014)

Department of Health (DH) (2001) *Valuing People: a new strategy for learning disabilities for the 21st Century.* HMSO, London.

Garvey, F. & Vincent, J. (2006) The bio-physical aspects of learning disabilities. *In* Peate, I. & Fearns, D. (2006) *Caring for People with Learning Disabilities.* Chichester, Wiley.

Gilbert, T. (2009) From the workhouse to citizenship: four ages of learning disability. *In* Jukes, M. (ed.) (2009) *Learning Disability Nursing Practice.* London, Quay Books.

Hallawell, B. (2009) Challenges for the curriculum in learning disability nursing. *In* Jukes, M. (ed.) (2009) *Learning Disability Nursing Practice.* London, Quay Books.

Heuser, S. (2012) The human condition as seen from the cross: Luther and disability. *In* Brock, B. & Swinton, J. (2012) *Disability in the Christian Tradition.* Cambridge, Eerdmans.

Jukes, M. (ed.) (2009) *Learning Disability Nursing Practice.* London, Quay Books.

Mencap (2011) *Shaping our Future: Mencap strategy 2011–2016.* Available at: www.mencap.org.uk/sites/default/files/documents/Mencap%20Strategy%202011_2016.pdf (last accessed 16 October 2014)

Newcastle University (2011) *Definition and Classification of Learning Disability*. Available at: http://tinyurl.com/BJHCAlearning1 (last accessed 16 October 2014)

New Scientist (2009) A rational alternative to testing IQ (editorial). *New Scientist*, 2 November. Available at: http://tinyurl.com/BJHCAlearning3 (last accessed 16 October 2014)

Office for National Statistics (ONS) (2011) www.ons.gov.uk/ons/taxonomy/index.html?nscl=Population (last accessed 16 October 2014)

Romero, M. (2012) Aquinas on the *corporis infirmitas*: broken flesh and the grammar of grace. *In* Brock, B. & Swinton, J. (2012) *Disability in the Christian Tradition*. Cambridge, Eerdmans.

03

NURSING SUPPORT FOR THOSE WITH PROFOUND AND MULTIPLE LEARNING DISABILITIES

AIMS AND LEARNING OUTCOMES:

The aims of this chapter are:

- To explore what profound and multiple learning disability (PMLD) is

- To highlight the areas of care that a person who has a PMLD is likely to express, experience and need meeting.

By the end of this chapter, the reader will be able to:

- Understand and discuss what PMLD is

- Have a basic understanding of the 'twelve activities of daily living' model of care

- Have a basic understanding of how these twelve activities of daily living could be applied when working with a person who has a PMLD.

INTRODUCTION

Chapter 2 highlighted a number of possible definitions and meanings of learning disability and suggested that the various meanings of learning disability are intimately bound up with the use of language and that as language changes, so does our understanding of those with a learning disability. It was suggested also that learning disability is a spectrum of conditions ranging from 'borderline' to 'profound'.

This chapter will highlight the needs and care of Thomas, a 65-year-old gentleman with a profound and multiple learning disability (PMLD) who has recently had a heart attack. Although Thomas lives in a small care home, he was admitted to an intensive care ward and then transferred to a medical ward of his local general hospital. Whilst set against the backdrop of a busy medical ward, the contents of this chapter will have value for those working in other hospital-based clinical areas, community services and care and nursing homes, as those with a PMLD are also likely to access these services or clinical areas.

This chapter will provide a simple 'definition' of what PMLD is, briefly explain one model of holistic care and then explore how this model of care can be applied to those with a PMLD.

SCENARIO 3.1

Thomas is a 65-year-old gentleman who lives within a social care home and has a profound and multiple learning disability (PMLD) with additional needs in the following areas:

- Severe mobility problems; is unable to sit without assistance and mobilise without the use of a wheelchair

- Pre-verbal communication skills; needs assistance to communicate

- Inability to digest food and drinks due to dysphagia; requires assistance to eat and drink

- Arthritis

- Epilepsy

- Pain management

- Taking and monitoring medication and their side-effects

- Doubly incontinent

- Personal hygiene; needs help with washing and bathing.

Thomas has suffered a heart attack and has been admitted to the ward on which Sally, the senior staff nurse introduced in *Chapter 1*, works.

WHAT IS PMLD?

What does profound and multiple learning disability (PMLD) mean? That is a fair question; after all, for some HCAs, student nurses and staff nurses, the whole idea of having a learning disability may be difficult to comprehend, let alone its various components or manifestations.

It is notoriously difficult to estimate with any precision the number of those with a PMLD in the UK. However, it is estimated that there are between 250 000 and 350 000 people in the UK who have a PMLD (Foundation for People with Learning Disabilities, 2005).

Those with a PMLD, as well as having a profound learning disability (as indicated by an IQ of less than 40), are likely to have more than one disability which could include:

- Neurological issues such as epilepsy
- Physical disabilities such as cerebral palsy which will impact on the person's mobility
- Significant communication, eating and drinking problems
- Respiratory and cardiovascular problems, sensory impairments, mental health issues, 'classic autism'
- Increased health problems that could be associated with any or all of the above.

Those with a PMLD are thus very likely to need significant additional support in order to maintain an optimum level of health and to engage within society.

TWELVE ACTIVITIES OF DAILY LIVING

In the past, as they are today, student nurses in all four pre-registration fields of practice were taught the vital importance of assessing the holistic needs of the patient or service user and then planning, implementing and evaluating a therapeutic and supportive care plan that met these assessed needs. This process of assessing, planning, implementing and evaluating care intervention was known as the 'nursing process'. This nursing process utilised the work of three nursing theorists (Nancy Roper, Winifred Logan and Alison Tierney): this work being the 'twelve activities of daily living' (ADLs) (Roper, Logan and Tierney, 1980; 2000).

The twelve activities of daily living are:

- Maintaining a safe environment
- Communication
- Breathing
- Eating and drinking
- Elimination
- Washing and dressing
- Controlling temperature
- Mobilisation
- Working and playing
- Expressing sexuality
- Sleeping
- Death and dying.

These twelve activities of daily living often served as a useful structure for patient or service user assessment and resultant care planning, usually within a hospital setting. However, mental health, neurological issues such as epilepsy, emotional care and spiritual care appeared to be missing from this particular care model and any holistic health care assessment and resultant care and support package must take these elements into account. As Thomas is likely to experience and express a need for a high level of support in virtually all areas of his life, this model of assessment and support will be utilised.

The role of the nurse

Within this current context, the first role of the nurse, nursing student and HCA is to reassure Thomas, who is likely to be anxious if not downright scared. Do not forget that Thomas is likely to be in pain and confused as he is in an unfamiliar environment and among people that he does not know. All of these are likely to increase his anxiety levels.

Their second priority is to assess holistically Thomas's needs with a 'strengths and needs' model, using the framework suggested by the twelve activities of daily living. Parts of this assessment may be relatively straightforward to complete and record, whilst other aspects may be less so. Do not forget to involve Thomas, any care staff from his care home and his family (if appropriate) in this assessment as much as possible, as not only will much useful information be gathered this way but it is also good practice. After all, if you (the reader) were a hospital patient, would you like your own care needs assessed and planned for without your involvement? Ideally, any care assessment and resultant care planning should be done on a multi-disciplinary basis, and this must include the views of the patient. Check and use any 'hospital pass-book' that may accompany Thomas, as this is likely to contain much useful information about Thomas's likes, dislikes and needs as well as how his needs are usually met. Any resultant care plans must likewise be holistic and incorporate Thomas's views, likes and dislikes.

Maintaining a safe environment

Thomas, along with everyone else, needs a safe environment in which to live. Maintaining a safe environment for Thomas is likely to include many of the following:

- Does Thomas have a history of falls, epilepsy or ear infections that may affect his balance?
- Does Thomas have any known allergies that could impact upon the care and support that he receives whilst in the hospital?
- Does Thomas require any specific manual handling equipment and if so, is this equipment such as hoists and slings regularly serviced and maintained?
- Does Thomas require mobility assistance, such as wheelchairs?
- Does Thomas require assistance to maintain healthy skin and prevent the occurrence of skin tissue breakdown such as pressure sores and ulcers?
- Does Thomas require any specific 'feeding equipment' such as percutaneous endoscopic gastrostomy (PEG) equipment in order to maintain optimum nutrition and if so, is this feeding equipment regularly cleaned, serviced and maintained?
- Are nursing and other care staff adequately and appropriately trained to use any equipment that Thomas needs to maintain optimum health?
- Is Thomas's immediate environment free from unacceptable and inappropriate risks, such as clutter?

Communication

Thomas has very little verbal communication skill and is limited to grunts, groans, cries and the occasional scream. Thomas communicates through facial expression, body language, basic Makaton and the occasional 'verbalisation'. Makaton is a sign language that was derived from British Sign Language and is used with and by people with a learning disability and, more recently, those with Alzheimer's dementia. Makaton is a language programme using signs and symbols to help people to communicate. It is designed to support spoken language and the signs and symbols are used with speech, in spoken word order (Makaton Charity, 2014).

Thomas has a variety of communication problems and needs (Griffiths and Doyle, 2009). These include making himself understood, understanding others, and having to rely on others to interpret what he is trying to say.

It is imperative that, at least initially, Sally take her cue from the care home staff that have accompanied Thomas. Once Sally gets to know Thomas, she should build upon her observations of Thomas and the way that he communicates with his care home staff and initiate conversations with him. Never forget, communication is a basic human right.

Breathing

As Thomas has had a heart attack, the quality and quantity of his respiration may be affected. This must be monitored and appropriate support offered. Thomas's posture may also impact negatively upon his ability to breathe properly. Therefore, the input of a physiotherapist or occupational therapist may be required to ensure that Thomas is sitting or lying correctly and that his posture is not impeding his ability to breathe.

Eating and drinking

Thomas, like many other people with a PMLD, experiences dysphagia (difficulty in swallowing) and requires all of his food and drink to be the consistency of a 'thickish' paste. This involves having his meals puréed and his drinks thickened with a proprietary thickener such as 'Thick & Easy'. It must never be forgotten, however, that the consumption of food and drink is not just a mechanical or bio-physical process as it involves the physical, emotional and psychological sensations of taste and touch, as well as incorporating socio-cultural and memory elements. Having a PMLD must not preclude Thomas from engaging in eating and drinking as social and cultural activities and experiences.

In order to maintain optimum nutritional levels and balance and for the optimum administration of medicines, the possibility of percutaneous endoscopic gastrostomy is being considered. For Thomas this is an endoscopic medical procedure in which a tube (PEG tube) is passed into a patient's stomach through the abdominal wall and through which nutrition/food, drinks and medicines will be passed (PEG feeding).

Elimination

"...Good morning Thomas. Oh, you've messed your bed again."

I know, it's not my fault and anyway I have had to lie in it for the last hour.

(paraphrased from Griffiths and Doyle, 2009, p. 285)

- How do you think Thomas feels at being told that he has messed his bed again?

- How do you think Thomas feels about not being checked, cleaned and changed before now?

Those with PMLD, like Thomas, are very likely to experience both urinary and fecal incontinence (Griffiths and Doyle, 2009). As a senior staff nurse, Sally is likely first of all to participate in the assessment of Thomas's continence levels and abilities and the impact that such incontinence has on the quality of Thomas's life.

Following this initial assessment, the resultant nursing care plan may include the following:

- Monitoring of the side-effects of any medicines that Thomas may be taking. All medicines have side-effects and some of these may affect his levels of urinary and fecal continence;
- Ensuring that any continence aids that Thomas normally uses at his care home continue to be used whilst on the hospital ward. This ensures continuity of care;
- Ensuring that any continence aids such as pads are used appropriately and correctly, are fit for purpose, fit Thomas comfortably, do not leak, are changed regularly and are not visible underneath his clothing;
- If appropriate and possible, encouraging Thomas to use 'ordinary' toilet facilities, bearing in mind that his mobility is decreased;
- Ensuring that Thomas's abilities and needs are reviewed regularly.

Washing and dressing

Thomas requires assistance with all aspects of personal hygiene, oral hygiene and dressing. This involves the choosing of cleaning and personal and oral hygiene products, the choosing and purchasing of clothing and choosing which items of clothing to wear on any given day. Thomas, being doubly incontinent, is likely to require extra assistance to maintain optimum personal hygiene. Such assistance must be offered gently, sensitively and with the utmost care and attention to detail, including privacy.

Controlling temperature

As Thomas is unable to tell you whether he is hot, cold or feels 'just right', let alone to control his own temperature, Sally will need to be aware of any subtle changes in his behaviour (whether, for example, he appears more agitated or aggressive or less engaged than usual), in facial expression and body language. Sally will also need to report and record these subtle changes as they form most of Thomas's communication repertoire, and then act upon them.

Such actions may involve:

- Offering to decrease or increase the amount of clothing that Thomas wears
- Increasing or decreasing the amount of bed covering (blankets) that Thomas has
- Increasing or decreasing the 'ambient' temperature through the use of small fans or portable heaters, if appropriate and safe.

The effects, if any, on Thomas's behaviour and how he communicates need to be monitored, reported and recorded.

Mobilisation

Thomas has profound mobility problems and is unable to walk. However, he is able to weight bear for very short periods of time and to stretch out his arms; these abilities must be encouraged and may be useful in helping Thomas to get dressed and undressed. The advice and support of Thomas's care home staff, the physiotherapist and the occupational therapist are likely to be essential to maximise Thomas's mobility capacity. Although unable to walk, Thomas does own and use a purpose-built wheelchair and this wheelchair must be maintained and utilised whilst he is on Sally's ward.

The physiotherapist would also be able to advise on a number of simple physical exercises that could prevent muscle and joint pain and keep his joints and limbs working and mobile.

Working and playing

It is unlikely that those with a PMLD are able to work in the same way and on the same basis that Sally is able to. It will be unrealistic for those with a PMLD to obtain and hold down a paid job in a shop, an office, a factory or on a hospital ward as an HCA or nurse. However, without being patronising or condescending, those with a PMLD are capable of engaging in a number of 'work-related' activities around the house and at any day care facilities that they may attend. Thomas, for example, enjoys assisting with the housework and the preparation of meals and cooking where he lives. This he does through holding the vacuum cleaner's hose pipe and pushing it across the floor, holding a duster and wiping the table tops and mixing food (such as a cake mixture) in a bowl or helping to make sandwiches. Thomas may need assistance to understand why he cannot engage in these activities whilst on Sally's hospital ward.

Thomas does enjoy going out shopping and for coffee, and accessing the countryside near where he lives. It may be appropriate for Thomas to be assisted to visit the hospital café or restaurant whilst he is in hospital.

Expressing sexuality

Of all the twelve ADLs, this is likely to be one of the two most contentious and difficult for nursing and other care staff to work with. Yet human sexuality is a crucial aspect of the human identity and what it means to be human. Thomas, despite having a PMLD, has the same sexual drives and needs as anyone else. However, expressing sexuality involves more than just the physical act of sex, as it also encompasses such diverse elements as clothing styles, use of cosmetics, hair styles, use of language, social and employment activities and even the music one listens to.

Sally's role is to:

- Understand how all these elements impact upon the person who is Thomas
- Be aware of and understand how Thomas expresses his sexuality
- Safeguard and promote his individual choices
- Ensure that his right to privacy is recognised, safeguarded and promoted.

Sleeping

Thomas experiences occasional problems in sleeping at night due, in part, to his tendency to sleep during the day because of under-stimulation and boredom, and his need to be turned regularly at night in order to prevent tissue breakdown. A number of issues need to be addressed here:

- Thomas's sleep pattern needs to be monitored. This must involve an assessment of both quantity and quality of sleep as well as Thomas's comfort (noise levels, whether he is too hot or cold and the suitability of the bed and mattress) and the actual timing of his sleep patterns
- Thomas needs to be kept fully engaged in social activities during the day
- Disruption to Thomas's night-time sleep pattern must be kept to a minimum
- Thomas's medication may need to be reviewed as insomnia may feature as a side-effect of some pre-existing medication and the introduction of 'night-time sedation' may need to be considered (although this is likely to be a last resort measure).

Death and dying

As with sexuality, death and dying is one of the two most contentious ADLs. Whilst Thomas shares this ultimate destiny with all of humanity and, indeed, with all living things, this is not to say that Thomas will die or is likely to, whilst in Sally's care. Nonetheless, the possibility of Thomas's death must be acknowledged and accepted.

Sally's roles are to reassure Thomas and explain to him what is happening in ways that he can understand and to liaise and work with other members of the hospital care team, including the hospital chaplaincy team if appropriate, Thomas's family and Thomas's care home staff, in relation to end of life care (whether these needs are perceived or actual).

CONCLUSION

As can be seen from the above, PMLD affects Thomas in virtually every aspect of his life. It is likely that, at some point in Sally's career as a staff nurse or nurse manager she will come into contact and work with patients like Thomas, so the aim of this chapter is to provide a small number of suggestions as to how Sally can work with and meet the needs of those with a PMLD within a hospital setting. However, be warned: the use of the 'twelve activities of daily living' and other similar assessment and care planning models are not to be used as a sterile 'tick box' activity, nor to be written in stone. Those with a PMLD deserve and have a right to better than that. Such models are to be seen and used as guidance for appropriate care assessment and planning only.

KEY POINTS

- It is estimated that there are between 250 000 and 350 000 people in the UK who have a PMLD.

- PMLD can be defined as having an IQ level of below 40 and with a wide range of additional physical, neurological and sensory disabilities.

- One of the models of care that may be useful in meeting the holistic care needs of those with a PMLD is the twelve activities of daily living devised by Roper, Logan and Tierney.

- Caution must be exercised in not turning this care model into a 'tick box' method of caring.

REFERENCES

Foundation for People with Learning Disabilities (2005) Available at: www. learningdisabilities.org.uk/page.cfm (last accessed 16 October 2014)

Griffiths, C. & Doyle, C. (2009) Nursing people with profound and multiple learning disabilities. *In* Jukes, M. (ed.) (2009) *Learning Disability Nursing Practice*. London, Quay Books.

Makaton Charity (2014) *About Makaton*. Available at: www.makaton.org/aboutMakaton/ (last accessed 16 October 2014)

Roper, N., Logan, W.W. & Tierney, A.J. (1980) *The Elements of Nursing*. Churchill Livingstone.

Roper, N., Logan, W.W. & Tierney, A.J. (2000) *The Roper–Logan–Tierney Model of Nursing: based on activities of living*. Edinburgh: Elsevier Health Sciences.

04

LEGISLATION, STRATEGIES AND REPORTS FOR THOSE WITH A LEARNING DISABILITY

AIMS AND LEARNING OUTCOMES:

The aims of this chapter are to highlight:

- The differences between the various forms of legislation and associated documents

- The various laws, White Papers and reports that have an impact specific to those with a learning disability

- A number of issues within these documents that have a specific impact upon nurses and nursing practice.

By the end of this chapter, the reader will be able to have a working knowledge of:

- The differences between a Parliamentary Bill, a Parliamentary Act, a Green Paper, a White Paper and an independent report

- The various pieces of legislation and associated documents that have a specific impact upon those with a learning disability

- How these various documents may impact upon their own nursing practice.

PAUSE FOR THOUGHT 4.1

Those who are not aware of and understand their history are condemned to repeat its mistakes: discuss!

INTRODUCTION

The area of health and social care law, Green Papers, White Papers and reports is both fascinating and complex. It can certainly be confusing and frustrating! Yet, not to have a working knowledge and understanding of these relevant Government documents that impact upon the lives of those with a learning disability could, and probably will, have serious consequences on the quality and forms of services that people with a learning disability receive. Understanding these government documents and policies will help you to both comply with the law and provide high-quality care to people with a learning disability.

It must be stated here that those who have a learning disability are subject to the same laws, both civil and criminal, as everyone else in society; having a learning disability does not exclude the person from the consequences, rights and responsibilities of the law and their conduct under the law, and neither should it! However, there are a number of laws that have a specific impact upon those with a learning disability and these will serve as the basis for this chapter.

Hanif (the 2nd year student nurse), Marcel (the young man who has Down's syndrome) and Ziva (Marcel's sister who also has high-functioning autism/Asperger's syndrome) have very kindly agreed to act as your guides throughout this chapter.

This chapter will highlight the contents and the impact of the wide variety of Parliamentary Bills, Parliamentary Acts, White Papers and reports that impact upon the lives of those with a learning disability over the past 40 years.

DIFFERENCES BETWEEN BILLS, ACTS, WHITE PAPERS, GREEN PAPERS AND REPORTS

It seems almost like every day that this, that or the other Bill, Act, report or whatever is released and highlighted in the daily newspapers, on radio and TV. There is no way that we, as members of society, can ignore such media attention and debate into what may often seem to be rather dry, obscure, obtuse and even apparently irrelevant issues. And neither should we. As nurses, as health care professionals we live and work in a legislation-rich environment and that is the way it has always been, always will be and indeed must be!

So, what is the difference between a Parliamentary Bill, a Parliamentary Act, a Green Paper, a White Paper and an independently commissioned report?

Marcel: Welcome to this brief highlighting of the various laws and reports that have such a huge effect on me and those like me. To be honest, I find that I can't quite get my head around much of these laws and reports and I am not alone here. Therefore, to a large extent I have to rely upon you, our reader, and your nursing and medical colleagues to be aware of, understand and implement these laws. So, again, welcome and let's continue. Ziva, my lovely sister, what is a Parliamentary Bill?

Ziva: Well, a *Parliamentary Bill* is an intended piece of legislation which originates from either the House of Lords or the House of Commons. Some Bills start life as part of the annual Queen's speech to Parliament and then become part of the Government's legislative programme whilst others are presented and sponsored by a backbench MP (any backbench MP can present and sponsor a Parliamentary Bill) or a member of the House of Lords. An example of the former could include the 'Care Bill 2013' and an example of the latter could include the 'Autism Bill 2009' which was sponsored by Cheryl Gillan (MP).

Marcel: So, how exactly does a Bill become law?

Ziva: Taking the 2009 Autism Bill as an example, its parliamentary journey included first and second readings, committee stage, report stage and third reading in the House of Commons. This process was then repeated in the House of Lords. The Autism Bill returned to the House of Commons where any amendments proposed by the Lords were debated and either accepted, amended or discarded. Once consensus had been reached by both Houses of Parliament, the Bill was presented to the Queen for signing. Once signed by the Queen (as Head of State), the Autism Bill became the Autism Act 2009.

Marcel: Thanks for that, sis! Hanif, how does a Bill differ from an Act?

Hanif: Well, a *Parliamentary Act* is a Parliamentary Bill that has successfully completed its parliamentary journey, been presented to and signed by the sovereign (the Queen or King), acting in her or his capacity as Head of State. Then, and only then, does it have any legal power and can be implemented. Some Parliamentary Acts serve to prohibit certain actions or behaviour of individual citizens or organisations whilst others permit certain actions or behaviour. An example of the former could include the Marine Broadcasting Offences Act 1967, which made illegal pirate radio stations such as Radio Caroline. An example of the latter could include the Abortion Act 1967, which permitted legal abortions under certain conditions.

Marcel: So, what are Green and White Papers?

Ziva: A *Green Paper* is a discussion or consultation document that is issued by political parties around specific issues such as mental health, transport or the environment, whereas a *White Paper* (such as *Valuing People* (DH, 2001)) is a policy document that is often published by the Government. One of the purposes of a White Paper is to present service delivery guidelines which, although not mandatory, would be very good practice if they were to be implemented.

Marcel: So, how do reports fit into all this?

Hanif: An Independent Report is a report into specific events or issues and is often written or commissioned by organisations, such as Mencap, that are outside of formal government structures. Examples of such reports could include *The Francis Report* 2013, Mencap's *Death by Indifference* (2007/2012) and the report into the abuse of people with a learning disability who were residents at Winterbourne View hospital in 2011. These independent reports often serve as a catalyst both for changes in how services are organised and delivered, and for the amendment or generation of new legislation.

Marcel: Thanks for this, Hanif and Ziva. I have a slightly better understanding of these various documents. Now, we will look at a number of these documents that have an impact upon me, those like me and those who are reading this.

BETTER SERVICES FOR THE MENTALLY HANDICAPPED (1971)

This White Paper came about partly as a result of a number of critical reports into the standard, type and quality of care that those with a learning disability received at a number of mental handicap (learning disability) hospitals in England and Wales. This report recommended halving the number of hospital places for those with a learning disability and that long-stay hospital settings for people with learning disabilities should gradually be closed and replaced with residential and 'day care' support in the community. Personal assessment of service user needs and greater involvement of the families of those with a learning disability were highlighted (Concannon, 2005).

Marcel: It took many years before many if not most of these recommendations became a reality for me and my friends.

JAY REPORT (1979)

The Jay Report was set up under the chairmanship of Mrs Peggy Jay. The Report called for a review of nurse training and proposed a new model that was more in line with the philosophy of ordinary living. However, the Report was critical of large institutional forms of service provision located on the edges of towns and cities and argued that such residential provision did not allow for community engagement. The Report argued that those with a mental handicap/learning disability had the right to live in an ordinary house in an ordinary street and to use and benefit from ordinary community resources. The framework of services should be one that both respects the person using the service and also meets the person's needs. Finally, the Report recommended that mentally handicapped adults should have residential provision in or near the social and geographical communities in which they spent their childhood or early adulthood (Concannon, 2005).

Marcel: Once again, the issue of where I was to live was prominent in this report, although the language used throughout was that of rights and choice. However, it is likely that most people like me would not have been asked to have contributed to this Report.

MENTAL HEALTH ACT 1983

The Mental Health Act was the first piece of mental health law since 1959.

Part 1/Section 1: sets out the legal definition of learning disability (mental and severe mental impairment) as being an 'arrested or incomplete development of mind which includes a significant or severe impairment of intelligence and social functioning'.

Part 2/Sections 2–5: allows for compulsory or voluntary admission to hospital either for assessment or treatment of a serious mental health issue. Section 5 allows doctors and mental health/learning disability nurses to prevent those with serious mental health issues from leaving a hospital. This section is applied if the patient is at high risk of harming themself or others if discharged from hospital.

Parts 3–5 deal with patients concerned in criminal proceedings or who are under sentence, consent to treatment (more on this in *Chapter 6*) and mental health tribunals.

NHS AND COMMUNITY CARE ACT 1990

The NHS and Community Care Act introduced an 'internal market' into the supply of health and social care within England, Scotland and Wales, with the State (local authorities) being more an 'enabler'/broker than a direct health and social care provider. Local authorities were tasked to take the lead in enabling social care assessment and provision. The Act restructured the NHS into NHS Trusts and included the establishment of 'fund-holding' GP practices.

The Act highlighted the rights of those with a learning disability to be active participating members of their local communities, living and working within that community (Kelly, 2006) and provided assistance to allow those with a learning disability to remain in their own homes should they wish (Fearns, 2006).

Marcel: At long last: ideas about how I am to be cared for and where I am to live that have been around for between 10–20 years have now found a home in law.

DISABILITY DISCRIMINATION ACT 1995

This Act made discrimination on the grounds of disability an offence. After defining what disability meant, the Act placed a duty on employers not to discriminate against employees or employment applicants on grounds of disability. In 1995, this applied to employers who employed more than 15 people. However, from 2004 onwards, the contents of this Act applied to all employers (McIver, 2006). The employer had a duty to make adjustments to the application and selection process and to the work premises and environment (including any equipment used by the employee).

Part 3 of the Act placed a duty on service providers such as banks, social and health care facilities, shops, restaurants/cafés, cinemas, theatres, pubs, hotels, art galleries and museums, railway stations, airports and faith community premises to provide appropriate and reasonable disability access to their premises and equality of treatment once on the premises.

Part 4 made it an offence to discriminate against or disadvantage pupils/students on the grounds of any disability that they may have. This applies to all educational environments and premises from nursery schools / crèches through to universities. This includes admission procedures, course content and teaching / assessment methods.

Part 5 gave the Government powers to make regulations relating to the design and accessibility of public transport, whilst Part 6 created the National Disability Council.

VALUING PEOPLE (2001)

This was the first White Paper that deals specifically with those with a learning disability for 30 years and comprised eleven key objectives, most of which will have a direct impact upon nursing care:

1. Maximising life opportunities for children with a learning disability through ensuring optimum access and use of educational, health and social care services whilst maintaining the child at home;
2. Transition into adult life through ensuring continuity of educational, health and social care and support for the young person and their family;
3. Enabling people to have more control and choice over their own lives through a person-centred approach to planning;
4. Increasing the help and support that the 'informal' care givers receive from local authorities;
5. Enabling people with learning disabilities to access a high-quality health service designed around their individual needs;
6. Enabling those with a learning disability and their families to have a greater choice of where and how to live;
7. Enabling people with learning disabilities to lead full and meaningful lives in their communities and to develop a range of friendships, activities and relationships;
8. Enabling more people with learning disabilities to make a valued contribution to the world of work through participating in all forms of paid employment;
9. Ensuring that all care agencies commission and provide high-quality, evidence-based, cost-effective and continuously improving services;
10. Ensuring that social and health care staff working with people with learning disabilities are appropriately skilled, trained and qualified;
11. To promote holistic services for people with learning disabilities through effective partnership working between all relevant local agencies in the commissioning and delivery of services.

MENTAL CAPACITY ACT 2005

Whilst the Mental Capacity Act 2005 will be highlighted and discussed more fully in *Chapter 6*, the brief summary below may be useful.

The Act promotes and safeguards the right to make decisions and to accept and refuse any health care, social care, nursing and medical interventions if the person has the capacity to do so. It also safeguards those who, for whatever reason, do not have mental capacity. The Act allows for advance decisions to refuse treatment and for the establishment of a 'lasting power of attorney' (someone who can decide and act on behalf of another person). It is imperative that any assessment of capacity and any decisions and interventions that are based on the assessment are recorded and reported.

DEATH BY INDIFFERENCE (MENCAP, 2007)

In March 2007, following the deaths of six people with a learning disability in NHS care, Mencap published 'Death by Indifference', which exposed the unequal healthcare and institutional discrimination that people with a learning disability often experienced within the NHS. Death by Indifference played an important role in influencing the Department of Health to commission the confidential enquiry into premature deaths of people with a learning disability. The Report called for learning disability liaison nurses to be established in all acute general hospitals to act as advisors to ward staff.

AUTISM ACT 2009

The Autism Act 2009 is the first disability-specific piece of law in the UK. The Act makes provision and offers guidance about meeting the needs of adults with autistic spectrum conditions on the part of local authorities and the NHS through the 'Autism Strategy'. Specific areas highlighted by this Act include diagnosing, identification and assessment of adults who are on the autism spectrum. The Act recommends holistic planning in relation to the provision of relevant services to people with autistic spectrum conditions as they move from being children to adults, and the training of staff who provide relevant services to adults with such conditions.

All local authorities are currently in the process of drafting local/regional autism strategies that meet and implement the above areas, many through local/regional autism partnership boards that comprise psychologists, psychiatrists, nurses, voluntary sector organisations, commissioners, parents and those on the autism spectrum.

EQUALITY ACT 2010

The Equality Act seeks to reduce socio-economic inequalities and eliminate discrimination and prohibit victimisation on a wide range of grounds including age, disability, gender, sexual orientation, marital status, ethnic background and religion and belief. The Act will prevent such discrimination through reasonable adjustments being made to service and premises access, access to education at all levels, employment selection and working conditions. For those who believe that they are discriminated against, remedies through the civil courts and employment tribunals are laid out.

DEATH BY INDIFFERENCE: 74 DEATHS AND COUNTING (MENCAP, 2012)

'*74 Deaths and Counting*' is a five-year review and progress report that is based on the Mencap report '*Death by Indifference*', published in 2007. Following on from the 2007 report, a further 68 deaths of those with a learning disability in general acute hospitals have come to light and a number of additional reports have been submitted:

- **2008**: *Healthcare for All: report of the independent inquiry into access to healthcare for people with learning disabilities*, Department of Health
- **2008**: *Six Lives*, Parliamentary and Health Service Ombudsman
- **2009**: *Valuing People Now*, Department of Health
- **2010**: *Six Lives Progress Report*, Department of Health

Issues that were highlighted in both the original 2007 and the current progress reports include lack of care for patients who have a learning disability, poor communication, failure to recognise pain, failure to monitor patients' health conditions, and diagnoses and treatment of health care conditions were delayed.

Do Not Resuscitate orders were made inappropriately, purely on the grounds of a patient having a learning disability, and the provisions and intentions of the Mental Capacity Act 2005 were routinely ignored. Doctors were rarely formally sanctioned or reprimanded by the General Medical Council (GMC) for these deaths.

Mencap made a number of recommendations including training for all health care professionals in relation to those with a learning disability, awareness of avoidable deaths and the identification and tracking of patients who have a learning disability whilst accessing health care services. Mencap suggested that family and other carers should be involved as a matter of course as partners in the provision of treatment and care. Finally, all Trust Boards should demonstrate in routine public reports that they have effective systems in place to deliver effective, 'reasonably adjusted' health services for those people who happen to have a learning disability.

CONCLUSION

This chapter has attempted to highlight a number of laws, White Papers and reports that have had a direct impact upon both the lives of those with a learning disability and on health care/service provision for this patient group over the past four decades. Understanding these government documents and policies is likely to prove rather challenging but may help you to comply with the law and to provide high quality care to people with a learning disability.

KEY POINTS

- There have been a number of pieces of legislation (Acts of Parliament/laws) and reports over the past 40 years that have had a direct impact upon the lives of those with a learning disability.

- Some of these have been as a direct result of a shift in thinking and attitudes towards those with a learning disability.

- Others have been as a direct result of poor quality nursing, medical and social care.

- The ultimate aim of these laws and reports is to improve the lives of those with a learning disability.

- The reading, understanding and implementation of these laws and reports are likely to prove challenging but worthwhile.

REFERENCES AND RESOURCES

Concannon, L. (2005) *Planning for Life: involving adults with learning disabilities in service planning*. Abingdon, Routledge.

Fearns, D. (2006) Protecting 'vulnerable' adults with learning disabilities. *In* Peate, I. & Fearns, D. (2006) *Caring for People with Learning Disabilities*. Chichester, John Wiley.

Kelly, J. (2006) Working with adults with learning disabilities. *In* Peate, I. & Fearns, D. (2006) *Caring for People with Learning Disabilities*. Chichester, John Wiley.

McIver, M. (2006) Legislation and learning disabilities. *In* Peate, I. & Fearns, D. (2006) *Caring for People with Learning Disabilities*. Chichester, John Wiley.

Mencap (2007) *Death by Indifference*. London, Mencap.

Mencap (2012) *Death by Indifference: 74 deaths and counting (a progress report 5 years on)*. London, Mencap.

Legislation

Autism Act 2009 www.legislation.gov.uk/ukpga/2009/15/contents

Disability Discrimination Act 1995 www.legislation.gov.uk/ukpga/1995/50/contents

Equality Act 2010 www.legislation.gov.uk/ukpga/2010/15/contents

Mental Capacity Act 2005 www.legislation.gov.uk/ukpga/2005/9/contents

Mental Health Act 1983 www.legislation.gov.uk/ukpga/1983/20/contents

National Health Service and Community Care Act 1990 www.legislation.gov.uk/ukpga/1990/19/contents

White Papers/reports

Department of Health (2001) *Valuing People: a new strategy for people with learning disabilities for the 21ˢᵗ Century.* Cm 5086. London, Department of Health.

Department of Health and Social Security/Welsh Office (1971) *Better Services for the Mentally Handicapped.* London, HMSO.

Jay, P. (1979) *The Report of the Committee of Enquiry into Mental Handicap Nursing and Care.* London, Department of Health.

Mencap (2007) *Death by Indifference.* London, Mencap.

Mencap (2012) *Death by Indifference: 74 deaths and counting.* London, Mencap.

05

MEDICAL CARE AND SUPPORT FOR THOSE WITH A LEARNING DISABILITY

AIMS AND LEARNING OUTCOMES:

The aims of this chapter are to:

- Highlight the support needs of those with a learning disability who access general health care facilities

- Highlight some of the barriers and issues that many people with a learning disability face whilst accessing health care services

- Set out a broad range of measures and interventions that could be put into place when working with this service user group within a 'general health care' setting such as a GP practice, a hospital ward or an outpatient department.

By the end of this chapter, the reader will have a working knowledge of:

- The care needs of a patient with a learning disability

- A number of barriers faced by those with a learning disability when they access health care facilities

- A number of measures and interventions that could be utilised to overcome these barriers.

INTRODUCTION

Many, if not most nurses, health care assistants and other health and social care professionals are likely, at some point in their work, to meet and provide general health care support and services to those with a learning disability within a number of health care settings. Such settings could include an Accident and Emergency (A&E) department, a general practice or health centre, an outpatient department, a surgical or medical ward or a dental practice. This chapter will focus on a number of practical issues that those with a learning disability may encounter when accessing such generalist health care services and settings.

How would you as a nurse, nursing student or health care assistant provide high-quality support to those with a learning disability within the environment where you work?

HEALTH CARE NEEDS OF THOSE WITH A LEARNING DISABILITY

SCENARIO 5.1

Ziva, a woman in her 30s who has high-functioning autism/Asperger's syndrome (HFA/AS) and is a university lecturer, and who also has a son with classic autism, is to be admitted to a gynaecological ward where Sally works as an occasional bank nurse, for a planned minor operation to remove uterine polyps by hysteroscopy.

SCENARIO 5.2

Marcel, a young man in his 30s with Down's syndrome who lives at home with his parents and is Ziva's brother, attends a pre-arranged 1 pm appointment at a local hospital's 'lumps and bumps clinic' (where, again, Sally works as an occasional bank nurse) for a large and painful cyst on his finger, having been referred to this clinic by his GP.

The Health of the Nation. A strategy for people with learning disabilities (Department of Health, 1995) recommended that:

"People with learning disabilities should have access to all general health services... with appropriate additional support as required to meet individual need... Any problems in obtaining health care for people with learning disabilities should be identified, and solutions found".

Those with a learning disability will experience the same health conditions and have the same health needs as everyone else. Many of these are relatively routine and commonplace such as the flu, chest and other infections, diabetes, health education, minor injuries, family planning and pregnancy, to name a few, and will be dealt with by the GP or practice nurse in the same way as anyone else but with additional support as and when needed. Other health conditions may require a more specialist medical or nursing input. Again, this is normal and is part and parcel of being human! Indeed, Barber (2001) made this clear in his paper on the professional development of nurses with regard to those on the autism spectrum. Although Barber's focus was on those with an autism spectrum condition, his point is applicable to those who have a learning disability.

However, many of those with a learning disability will experience specific health conditions. For example, respiratory, circulatory and cardiac problems are often associated with people who have Down's syndrome (National Association for Down's syndrome, 2010). Again, prevalence of epilepsy is often higher in those with a learning disability than elsewhere in society (Epilepsy Action, 2010). Likewise, there appears to be a higher incidence of mental health problems in those with a learning disability (RCN, 2010).

In previous decades, most relatively minor health care interventions for those with a learning disability were carried out within the old mental handicap hospitals. By 'relatively minor' is meant the type of health care issues one would usually see the GP, community nurse, optician or dentist about. Indeed, such hospitals tended to be very self-contained and provided more or less everything that the person with a learning disability needed. However, with the closure of these large and often isolated hospitals during the 1980s and 1990s, the provision of health care services was transferred to mainstream acute and community health care providers.

ROLES OF THE NURSE

There are a number of specific practical suggestions that could be useful to nurses, HCAs, student nurses and other health and social care professionals when working within a 'generalist' health care setting. Such settings are likely to include a GP practice or community health centre, an A&E or 'out of hours' unit, an outpatient unit or a surgical or medical ward. Some of the following practical suggestions may be more useful than others, whilst some may be easier to implement and may be cheaper to act upon than others. However, quality must never be sacrificed in order to keep down costs. Do not forget that the framework suggested by the 'twelve activities of daily living' in order to provide high-quality holistic care, highlighted in *Chapter 3*, could be useful here.

PAUSE FOR THOUGHT 5.2

What do you consider to be the steps required to ensure that Ziva and Marcel are admitted 'hassle free' to the ward or department where Sally works?

Access the support of the learning disability liaison nurse

In order to provide better support for both Marcel and Ziva during their stay at the hospital, a learning disability liaison nurse (LDLN) would be invaluable. An LDLN is a specialist learning disability trained nurse who supports people with a learning disability while they are in hospital to make sure they get the care they need.

Where there is an LDLN, it's important that they meet the patient as soon as possible after they arrive at the hospital. This is so that the LDLN can find out everything they need to know about the patient's learning disability and health condition and the help they will need while in hospital. It may be possible to arrange a meeting before the hospital stay.

The learning disability liaison nurse can assist with:

- Co-ordination of care – at points of attendance, admission and discharge
- Education within clinical areas and contributing to programmes of education
- Support and advice for acute care staff in relation to personalised care and service delivery
- Collaboration between the agencies involved in service delivery to ensure effective seamless care by undertaking home visits
- Development and enhancement of standards of care for all patients with a learning disability attending the acute hospital
- Promotion of effective communication with those involved in the patient's care – whether they are community or hospital based
- Support of a relative or a family member with a learning disability who is affected by the patient's illness / hospital stay
- Promoting safety and minimising risk
- Provision of accessible information about treatments
- Promotion of positive experiences and outcomes (NHS Lothian, 2013).

Assess, assess and assess

This may, perhaps, sound obvious but it is imperative that every service user or patient who has a learning disability must be treated as an individual. It may, therefore, not be appropriate to approach, assess or treat:

- a young child with a learning disability in exactly the same way as you would a teenager or an adult with a learning disability, or
- a person with severe or profound learning disability in the same way as a person with a mild or moderate learning disability

as each of these will have differing information, care and support needs. Therefore, not only must the patient assessment be absolutely thorough but it must be holistic, appropriate to the individual and fit for purpose. It may be necessary to devise a new set of health care assessments that meet the communication needs of those with a learning disability, if such do not exist where Sally works. For example, it may be necessary to substitute words and numerical scales with simple line drawings or pictures. One such example could be the pain scale developed by Jackson *et al.* (2006) where pictures of happy and sad faces are used to denote levels of pain.

Accessible information

It is vital for the service user or patient with a learning disability to have information that is simple, easy to understand, timely, accurate, and in a format that the patient can use. Although Ziva works as a university lecturer, the manner in which she processes information, particularly when stressed, may require such information to be presented in ways other than written or verbal. As the information levels and needs will vary from person to person and from condition to condition and even from day to day, the type and level of information that is offered will likewise have to vary, as will the ways in which this information is presented. Such communication issues will be highlighted during assessments. It is important, here, to be imaginative and creative in how appropriate information is offered, particularly within tight financial and time constraints. However, what must be borne in mind when providing information to people with a learning disability is that without appropriate information the patient's or service user's ability to give *informed* consent to treatment will be threatened and may even not exist. This could have potentially profound practical, legal and ethical consequences for both the patient and the nursing and medical staff.

Communication

Communication is the central key, the linchpin to everything that the nurse does with the patient or service user and is essential in order to gain consent to any intervention or care (Mental Health Foundation, 1996; Hart, 1998). It must be borne in mind that communication is not a one-way process (e.g. from nurse to patient) but is an active multi-way process involving a minimum of two people but likely to involve many more. However, the person with a profound learning disability, such as Thomas from *Chapter 4*, may either be totally non-verbal, may communicate through facial expressions and other forms of body language, through pre-verbal 'grunts' or through sign languages such as Makaton (a simpler form of British Sign Language). Therefore, it is vital for Sally to take the time and really observe, to really get to know the patient so that she can pick up on the various but hidden nuances in their behaviour, facial expressions and body language in order to ascertain what it is they are communicating.

In order to communicate, particularly with those who may be 'less-abled', imagination may be needed in order to present or acquire information and even to say 'Hello, how are you?' or to talk about the weather, TV programmes or the fact that a few years ago Southend United beat Manchester United 1:0!

Pre-admittance visits

PAUSE FOR THOUGHT 5.3

How would you arrange a pre-admittance visit by Ziva onto the ward on which Sally works?

Although this may not be possible, arranging pre-admittance visits for patients who have a learning disability may be very useful in order to familiarise that person with the routines, procedures, sights, sounds, smells and people within a hospital ward, outpatient department or dental surgery. Cumella and Martin (2000) cite examples of hospitals arranging such visits, recording video footage of 'life on a hospital ward' for those with a learning disability or preparing very simple pre-admittance information sheets and leaflets using a combination of actual photos, pictures and line drawings.

However, such pre-admittance visits can be resource-intensive and prohibitive in terms of money and time and in an environment that is increasingly budget-conscious, it may be difficult to justify such resources for what could be a relatively small number of patients. Having said that, do contact and talk to the learning disability liaison nurse for advice on how to produce accessible pre-admittance information. Also, by using relatively scarce resources in an imaginative and creative manner, it may be possible to produce simple and cheap information and short DVDs for those with a learning disability. Finally, the Mencap website (www.mencap.org.uk/) may provide useful suggestions regarding pre-admittance visits and information.

Timing of appointments

SCENARIO 5.2 CONT'D

Marcel, a young man in his 30s with Down's syndrome, attended a pre-arranged 1 pm appointment at a local hospital's 'lumps and bumps clinic' for a large and painful cyst on his finger, having been referred to this clinic by his GP. When Marcel arrived at this clinic, there were about a dozen other people waiting to be seen. A notice appeared on the clinic wall advising the patients that there was a 50 minute delay, which stretched to 55 and then 60 minutes. Marcel did not understand the delay or the reason for it and rapidly became agitated and anxious. Marcel started to pace up and down the waiting area, becoming more verbally and then physically agitated and aggressive, scratching and biting himself on his arms. The clinic staff asked the hospital security to escort Marcel out of the clinic and the hospital, saying that his behaviour was disruptive and was scaring other patients. Consequently, because Marcel was not seen by the clinic, his cyst was not diagnosed at this appointment as being pre-cancerous, which it actually was.

PAUSE FOR THOUGHT 5.4

How would you support Marcel in this particular situation?

Many of those with a learning disability, particularly those who are also on the autism spectrum, will have set and rigid daily routines which, if disrupted, may result in a 'behaviour meltdown'. Again, many of those with a learning disability will experience anxiety and stress and perhaps extreme anxiety if exposed to unfamiliar environments, smells and sounds and unexplained delays. Thus, it is important to keep disruption and resultant anxiety to an absolute minimum. One way to achieve this is to schedule medical appointments for fairly quiet times, either very early appointments or the last appointments of the day, so that there are fewer people around and lower noise levels which will lead to lower levels of sensory stimulation and arousal. If Marcel or Ziva need to visit the GP practice, health centre or outpatient department for any reason it may also be helpful to book a 'double appointment' in order to allow time for information to be given to the patient and for the patient to be able to ask questions regarding their health and treatment.

It would be very helpful if Marcel and Ziva could have any GP appointments with the same GP at each appointment. This would allow the GP and the patient to get to know each other and the patient would not feel that they have to repeat themselves to different doctors whom they see. It would certainly be helpful not to have a 'general appointment time' but, instead, to have specific appointment times. A nine o'clock appointment must mean 09.00 and not 09.30 or 10.00. This is less likely to heighten anxiety levels with a resultant 'behavioural meltdown' such as was experienced and expressed by Marcel. If appointments are delayed significantly for any reason, and in the real world this may very likely be the case, ongoing explanations for the delay and reassurance using language and terms that the patient with a learning disability is likely to understand, would be useful. As with Marcel, it may be helpful to lead the patient into a quiet room or area or to allow the patient to 'jump the queue'.

Personal 'passbooks'

PAUSE FOR THOUGHT 5.5

What, if anything, is wrong about the following question: *"Does he take sugar?"*

According to Cumella and Martin (2000), several hospitals are implementing patient-written and -held 'communication passports', which include the following information:

- A photograph of the person
- Information about key contacts and health needs
- The patient's likes and dislikes
- How they communicate
- Any dietary needs and food allergies
- Mobility issues
- Personal care issues
- Personal faith community contacts if needed
- Any medication that is being taken.

If nurses and HCAs are familiar with and read such passbooks, the need to ask whether the patient takes sugar in his tea or coffee becomes largely redundant.

Or does it? As a way of starting a conversation with a patient who has a learning disability, it may be useful to ask the patient if he or she has sugar in their coffee or tea. Marcel says that the point here is that the question should become "*Do you take sugar?*" rather than "*Does he take sugar?*". Marcel would very much prefer it if Sally or Hanif were to talk *to* him, not at or about him! However, those with a learning disability may not be able to verbally communicate, thus it is imperative to read their passbook and communicate with them in ways that they can understand and participate in.

Each hospital is likely to have its own version of this type of passbook but the format of using simple language and pictures to present information is likely be very similar. This passbook will be completed by the person with a learning disability or by someone who knows this person well. If such a passbook does not exist where Sally works, it may be worth contacting the learning disability liaison nurse for advice on how to design and produce one.

Support during admittance

Ziva

It may be helpful for Ziva to receive a text message the day before her appointment to remind her. Ziva, who was accompanied to the hospital by her husband, could be met at the hospital entrance by a 'buddy'. Such a 'buddy' could be arranged by the hospital's LDLN and may well be a volunteer. The role of the 'buddy' will be to explain to Ziva where her ward is and to take her there, to explain hospital and ward procedures and layout and to be a 'friendly face' in what can often be seen as a hostile and frightening environment.

Once on the ward, a full medical history and assessment that is relevant to the procedure must be taken. Ziva must be fully involved in the assessment, being treated as a person and not as a medical condition. As part of this assessment, Ziva's mobility and self-care abilities will be considered. As Ziva is articulate and is able to communicate verbally, it was felt that a passbook was not needed. However, due to her Asperger's syndrome Ziva asked for information to be offered initially using simple rather than complex language and jargon. Ziva was offered the opportunity to ask questions, questions which were answered honestly. Ziva was asked if she would like a side room as this was more likely to afford her quietness and may be less stressful for her.

Marcel

Marcel was fully able to communicate with the hospital staff at the outpatients clinic that he attended. However, the clinic staff failed to communicate effectively with him and this caused Marcel a lot of anxiety and resulted in 'inappropriate behaviour' on his part, which resulted in him being unable to attend his initial appointment. However, the hospital-based

LDLN was able to intervene at the request of Marcel's parents and Marcel was offered another appointment at the clinic. During this second appointment, Marcel was supported by the liaison nurse and his parents.

Support before the procedure

As the associate nurse for Marcel and Ziva, Sally discussed with them the various options for their respective conditions (it is more likely that the permanent rather than the bank staff would act as the named nurse). With Ziva, the option was having her polyps removed by hysteroscopy under either local or general anaesthetic. Sally assessed Ziva's ability to process and understand information and explained to her what this procedure actually entailed in terms that she was able to understand. Sally gave Ziva an information leaflet on the procedure and then left her to read it, returning to answer any questions that she may have had.

Marcel was offered and accepted support from the LDLN during his second appointment. The liaison nurse worked with Sally to ensure that Marcel was made aware of any delays in being seen and the reasons for these delays, and that Marcel was reassured.

Support during the procedure

Ziva was offered the choice between having the polyps removed under local or general anaesthetic and chose the former. As Ziva was conscious throughout, the procedure was explained to her step by step whilst her husband was given the option of using the staff room and having welcome cups of coffee whilst he waited for her to return to the ward. Marcel was supported by the LDLN throughout his second appointment at the 'lumps and bumps' clinic. It was suggested to Marcel that because of the small risk of the cyst being cancerous, a biopsy would be advisable. The liaison nurse explained to Marcel and his parents what this meant and would involve. Biopsy is a medical procedure where a sample of tissue is taken, usually under local or topical anaesthesia, for examination and diagnosis of an illness or medical condition such as cancer.

Support after the procedure

After the polyps were removed, Ziva was taken back to the side room on the gynaecology ward and was offered pain relief, verbal reassurance and careful monitoring. Any questions that Ziva had about the polyps and the procedure were answered by her named nurse.

After the excision of the cyst for biopsy, Marcel was given pain relief, an explanation of what would happen next, reassurance and a follow-up appointment.

Discharge

Given that discharge planning should commence when the patient is admitted onto the ward or department and should not be seen as an afterthought at the end of the stay, the key to a successful discharge for both Ziva and Marcel is communication, team working and appropriate referrals. As the associate nurse for Ziva, Sally was likely to be involved in drawing up her discharge plan. Ziva must be offered information about general gynaecology as well as condition-specific aftercare in a format that she can access and understand, taking into account any communication and information processing issues that may affect those with Asperger's. Ziva was reminded of the importance of having someone at home to look after her for a day or two. Ziva replied that her husband would be taking time off work to look after her. Ziva will be referred back to her GP for general check-ups and the results of tests that were carried out on the removed polyps, as some polyps may be cancerous in nature.

Marcel's discharge plan was likewise thorough. Marcel and his parents were offered easy to read information about the aftercare of a person who has had a cyst biopsy. A follow-up appointment was made during which the results of the cyst biopsy would be explained. As a result of the biopsy, a referral to a cancer specialist was made.

Follow-up

Ziva: 'Three weeks after I left the hospital, I received a phone call from the hospital learning disability liaison nurse enquiring how I was and how the follow-up appointments with my GP went. I thought that was a nice touch'.

Marcel: 'I was also contacted by the learning disability liaison nurse. I was visited at home by the dietician, the physiotherapist and the community learning disability nurse who liaised with the cancer specialists at the hospital. The community learning disability nurse ensured that I was resting and was looking after myself properly. He also arranged for any further health checks to be made'.

Professional development opportunities

According to Mencap there are continuing failures in care for people with a learning disability (Mencap, 2010). Since March 2007 when Mencap published '*Death by Indifference*' further deaths have been reported to Mencap, deaths which families blame on hospital blunders, *poorly trained staff* and indifference (Mencap, 2010). There is thus a need for nurses at all levels to receive awareness raising and basic training in learning disability care as part of their ongoing professional development programmes. It may be useful to contact either the local or regional Mencap office or the hospital-based LDLN for advice and suggestions as to how to access appropriate training that would cover the issues of what learning disability is and is not, as well as how to provide high-quality care to a patient who has a learning disability.

CONCLUSION

Those with a learning disability are as likely as anyone else to experience health issues and illnesses that require either the support of community-based health care such as GP practices or admittance to a general hospital. Nurses' knowledge about learning disability care is historically not as good as it should be and this has contributed to the needless deaths in general hospitals that resulted in the 2007 Mencap report *'Death by Indifference'*. However, those with a learning disability have a right to high-quality health, medical and nursing care and there is much that the nurse, student nurse and HCA working within a 'generalist' health care setting could do to ensure that high-quality care is delivered.

KEY POINTS

- Those with a learning disability are as likely to experience health issues and illnesses as anyone else.

- Historically, nurses and HCAs working in general health care settings are not trained to work with those who have a learning disability.

- There are a number of ways that hospital and community-based nurses could improve the quality of the nursing support experienced by those with a learning disability whilst accessing health care facilities.

- These include carrying out holistic assessments, providing appropriate information, pre-admission visits, timing of appointments, patient-held information 'passbooks' and communication.

REFERENCES

Barber, C. (2001) The training needs of registered nurses engaged in work with people with an autistic spectrum disorder. *Good Autism Practice*, 2:2; 86–96.

Cumella, S. & Martin, D. (2000) *Secondary Healthcare for People with a Learning Disability*. London, Department of Health.

Department of Health (DH) (1995) *The Health of the Nation. A strategy for people with learning disabilities*. London, HMSO.

Epilepsy Action (2010) *Learning Disabilities and Epilepsy*. Available at: www.epilepsy. org.uk/info/learning-disabilities/link-with-epilepsy (last accessed 16 October 2014)

Hart, S. (1998) Learning-disabled people's experience of general hospitals. *British Journal of Nursing*, 7, 470–477.

Jackson, D., Horn, S., Kersten, P. & Turner-Stokes, L. (2006) Development of a pictorial scale of pain intensity for patients with communication impairments: initial validation in a general population. *Clinical Medicine*, 6:6, 580–585.

Mencap (2010) *Needless Deaths Continue*. Available at: www.mencap.org.uk/news/article/needless-deaths-continue (last accessed 16 October 2014)

Mental Health Foundation (1996) *Building Expectations: opportunities and services for people with a learning disability*. London, Mental Health Foundation.

National Association for Down's Syndrome (2010) *Facts about Down Syndrome*. Available at: www.nads.org/pages_new/facts.html (last accessed 16 October 2014)

NHS Lothian (2013) *Acute Hospital Liaison Service*. Available at: www.nhslothian.scot.nhs.uk/Services/A-Z/LearningDisabilities/ClinicalServices/Pages/AcuteHospitalLiaisonService.aspx (last accessed 16 October 2014)

Royal College of Nursing (RCN) (2010) *Mental Health Nursing of Adults with Learning Disabilities*. Available at: www.rcn.org.uk/__data/assets/pdf_file/0006/78765/003184.pdf (last accessed 16 October 2014)

LEARNING DISABILITY AND CONSENT TO TREATMENT

The aims of this chapter are to:

- Define and discuss what consent is

- Discuss the issue of implied consent

- Highlight and discuss the contents of the Mental Capacity Act (MCA) 2005

- Highlight and discuss the nurse's role in consent and the applications of the MCA in relation to caring for someone who has a learning disability.

By the end of this chapter you will have a basic understanding of:

- What consent is and is not

- The contents of the Mental Capacity Act 2005

- How the MCA can be applied to those with a learning disability within a hospital setting.

SCENARIO 6.1

Marcel, a young man with Down's syndrome, arrives at the local Accident & Emergency (Casualty) department where Hanif works as a student nurse. Marcel was involved in a road traffic accident and, as a result, sustained a broken arm and leg. Marcel, who is unconscious, is accompanied by his sister Ziva who has Asperger's syndrome/high-functioning autism.

INTRODUCTION

Consent to treatment, indeed consent to any form of nursing, medical or social intervention, is a very complex issue and involves a wide range of professional, philosophical, legal and ethical questions and concerns. Registered nurses, student nurses and health care assistants will, in the course of a normal working day, have to assist patients or service users to make a myriad choices and decisions encompassing much of their daily lives whilst in their care. On occasion they may even have to either decide or contribute to the decision to provide nursing input as the patient is unable to decide for him- or herself. This may be for a wide range of reasons, including being unconscious, intoxicated through alcohol or other 'recreational' drugs or being in severe physical, mental or emotional pain. This is to be expected.

Likewise, nursing and other care staff are likely to encounter and work with people who have a learning disability who, due to their learning disability, are going to need extra support in making choices and decisions.

WHAT IS CONSENT?

Do we know what consent is? Yes? No? Maybe? Following on from this initial question, a number of subsequent questions spring to mind: Consent *to* and *for* what? Consent *by* whom? Consent *for* whom?

These are all valid and relevant questions and a lot of discussion by and between ethicists, philosophers, lawyers, nursing and medical practitioners, patients/service users and even theologians has taken place over the years in order to attempt to answer these and similar questions. Sometimes, however, it is likely that such debates have not led to consensus between the various stakeholders; this lack of consensus has had consequences for both patients/service users and hands-on clinical staff.

So, what is consent? Put simply, consent refers to the provision of approval or agreement between two or more people or between a person and an organisation, particularly and especially after thoughtful consideration, for an action to take place. According to the Oxford English Dictionary, consent is "the voluntary agreement to or acquiescence by one person in what another person proposes or desires". In other words, say Hobden and Mills (2008), within a health care setting "consent is permission by a patient or service user for health care professionals to touch, question, examine or deliver care to the patient or service user". Consent can either be verbal, gestural or written. Without such consent, any form of nursing, medical or social care intervention could be seen as a form of abuse.

For consent to be valid, the following criteria must be met. The consent has to be based on sufficient relevant information, voluntary and given by somebody who is capable of giving consent.

For Marcel, as for everyone else, information must be in a format and manner that can be readily understood. Such information could be presented as:

- Visual images such as pictures, line drawings and photos
- Spoken words using simple language and short sentences
- Leaflets, again using simple language and short and simple sentence structure
- Sign language such as Makaton
- A combination of these.

Information needs and the ways that such information is presented are likely to change over time and even from situation to situation.

Consent must be voluntary. This is even more relevant when a person is vulnerable or placed in a vulnerable position, such as having a learning disability, experiencing mental ill-health, experiencing acute pain, being the recipient of bad news, being under the influence of alcohol or other 'recreational drugs' or being unconscious. Care must be taken to ensure that consent is not obtained through coercion, bullying or the offering of 'inducements'. Such a situation is likely to be seen as abusive and any 'consent' obtained is likely to be invalid.

Those with a learning disability (such as Marcel) and/or those with a mental health issue must not be deemed unable to give or withhold consent purely on the grounds of their learning disability or mental health issue. There are strict criteria for assessing a person's mental capacity and ability to give consent; more about this later.

Remember, those who give consent for any form of medical or nursing intervention also have the legal and moral right to refuse to give consent or to withdraw consent at any time for a good reason, a bad reason or for no reason at all, and this right must be upheld.

FORMS OF CONSENT
Express consent

Express consent is where the patient articulates consent to a proposed course of action, either verbally, through gestures or in writing. In a more structured setting such as pre-operation, consent is usually recorded in writing using a pre-printed form. However, a problem may arise where there is a dispute between the patient and the care professional around the contents of any verbal consent. Here, what was said may come down to the 'patient's word' as opposed to that of the health care professional (Hobden and Mills, 2008). Never forget that the patient has a right to refuse to give consent or to withdraw consent once consent has been given.

In purely legal terms, there is no real difference between written and verbal consent and one form is not superior to the other (Hobden and Mills, 2008). However, the more complex the medical or surgical procedure, the more complex the information that the patient needs and thus the consent that is required.

Implied consent

Implied consent is no consent at all: discuss.

Marcel is now conscious and has been admitted to the ward on which Sally works as a part-time senior staff nurse. During the morning drug round Sally approaches Marcel without saying anything about medication and he holds his hand out. Is this Marcel consenting to the receiving and taking of medication or is it learned behaviour?

Implied consent is where the patient's *behaviour* indicates that he or she is giving consent to whatever intervention is being proposed. This could include:

- Marcel holding out his hand when Sally approaches him with his medicines during a drug round
- A person arriving at the A&E department where his presence at the department implies consent to nursing and/or medical intervention
- A patient at a GP practice blood test clinic rolling his sleeve up in readiness to having a blood sample taken, although the GP or practice nurse may not have asked him to do so.

However, be very careful here. Consent, be it expressed or implied, must not be taken as a blanket permission that covers all forms of treatment, intervention or procedure throughout the patient's stay at the hospital, health care clinic or GP surgery. If Marcel arrives on the ward where Sally works with an overnight bag, Sally and her colleagues must not take this as implied consent for major invasive surgical procedures – unless, of course, he is booked in for such procedures. Again, consent is not a 'one-off' event but is a dynamic phenomenon and process and must be sought and given for each intervention or treatment that is proposed.

One danger with implied consent is that healthcare professionals may make assumptions about the patient's willingness to consent based upon their current or previous actions or behaviours. Therefore, it is advisable to always check with the patient as to whether or not they are giving consent.

MENTAL CAPACITY ACT 2005

According to McIver (2006), the Mental Capacity Act (MCA) 2005 (originally the Mental Incapacity Bill), which affects everyone over the age of 16 years whose mental capacity 'is in doubt, is one of the most controversial pieces of legislation that relates to people with a learning disability'. Mental capacity, in relation to the MCA, refers to the ability of the individual to make a decision about a number of aspects of their lives, such as the ability to understand information and give fully informed consent, withdraw or withhold such consent. This would be the case not only in any health care setting but in other areas of life as well.

In its introductory paragraph, the MCA states that it is

'... an Act to make new provision relating to persons who lack capacity; to establish a superior court of record called the Court of Protection in place of the office of the Supreme Court called by that name; to make provision in connection with the Convention on the International Protection of Adults signed at the Hague on 13th January 2000; and for connected purposes'

(www.legislation.gov.uk/ukpga/2005/9/introduction)

So, how would the Mental Capacity Act 2005 impact upon Marcel throughout his stay at hospital following his road traffic accident? Remember that when Marcel first entered the hospital following his accident, he was unconscious and that when he was transferred to Sally's ward he was conscious. Therefore, his mental capacity, his ability to understand information and give, withhold or withdraw informed consent has changed, and will change over time.

The stated aims of the Mental Capacity Act 2005 are to provide a statutory framework that will empower and protect vulnerable people who are unable to make their own decisions and to make clear who can take decisions on behalf of another person and in what circumstances.

McIver (2006) suggests that:

'Individual care plans will have to conform to the principles of the Act, demonstrating that service users have either been involved in decisions about their care, or that they have been assessed as lacking the capacity to do so and that the decisions made are in their best interests'.

(McIver (2006), p. 154)

What the Act says

The Mental Capacity Act 2005 is split up into three separate parts:

Part 1: Contains 44 separate sections and focuses on people who may not possess mental capacity to make decisions or may have fluctuating ability.

Part 2: Focuses on the Court of Protection and the Public Guardian.

Part 3: Deals with miscellaneous and general issues.

There are, in addition, eleven 'Schedules' which focus on specific issues such as deprivation of liberty and lasting power of attorney.

It is likely that Part 1 of the MCA will be the most applicable to those who engage on a daily basis with people who have a learning disability.

Section 1 of the MCA: The principles

This introduces the five key principles that apply throughout the MCA:

- A person must be assumed to have capacity unless it is established that he lacks capacity

- A person is not to be treated as unable to make a decision (*such as to give, refuse or withdraw consent*) unless all practicable steps to help him to do so have been taken without success

- A person is not to be treated as unable to make a decision merely because he makes an unwise decision

- An act done, or decision made, under the *MCA* for or on behalf of a person who lacks capacity must be done, or made, in his or her best interests

- Before the act is done, or the decision is made, regard must be had to whether the purpose for which it is needed can be as effectively achieved in a way that is less restrictive of the person's rights and freedom of action.

(www.legislation.gov.uk/ukpga/2005/9/section/1)

Section 2 of the MCA: People who lack capacity

1. For the purposes of this Act, a person lacks capacity in relation to a matter if at the material time he is unable to make a decision for himself in relation to the matter because of an impairment of, or a disturbance in the functioning of, the mind or brain.

2. It does not matter whether the impairment or disturbance is permanent or temporary.

3. A lack of capacity cannot be established merely by reference to

   a. a person's age or appearance, or

   b. a condition of his, or an aspect of his behaviour, which might lead others to make unjustified assumptions about his capacity.

Section 2 of the MCA: People who lack capacity (cont'd)

4. In proceedings under this Act or any other enactment, any question whether a person lacks capacity within the meaning of this Act must be decided on the balance of probabilities.

5. No power which a person ("D") may exercise under this Act is exercisable in relation to a person under 16

   a. in relation to a person who lacks capacity, or

   b. where D reasonably thinks that a person lacks capacity.

(www.legislation.gov.uk/ukpga/2005/9/section/2)

McIver (2006) suggests that, under Section 2, the individual patient, such as Marcel, does not have to prove that he or she has mental capacity, no more than under the English justice system a person has to prove his or her innocence. Again, each assessment of Marcel's capacity to make decisions must be time- and issue-specific. By this is meant that an assessment of capacity must be done every time that a decision has to be made and for every decision.

Section 3 of the MCA: Inability to make decisions

1. For the purposes of Section 2, a person is unable to make a decision for himself if he is unable to:

   a. understand the information relevant to the decision

   b. retain that information

   c. use or weigh that information as part of the process of making the decision

   d. communicate his decision (whether by talking, using sign language or any other means).

2. A person is not to be regarded as unable to understand the information relevant to a decision if he is able to understand an explanation of it given to him in a way that is appropriate to his circumstances (using simple language, visual aids or any other means)

3. The fact that a person is able to retain the information relevant to a decision for a short period only does not prevent him from being regarded as able to make the decision

Section 3 of the MCA: Inability to make decisions (cont'd)

4. The information relevant to a decision includes information about the reasonably foreseeable consequences of:

   a. deciding one way or another, or

   b. failing to make the decision.

   (www.legislation.gov.uk/ukpga/2005/9/section/3)

However, McIver (2006) suggests that 'failure alone to understand the relevant information is not sufficient to demonstrate a lack of mental capacity'; Marcel is therefore not to be treated as unable to make decisions regarding his medical and nursing care simply because he makes an unwise decision. Section 4 will be highlighted in the next section.

There are a number of important sections of the MCA that will impact upon nursing care and support for Marcel and others with a learning disability whilst accessing health care:

- **Sections 9–14 and 22–23**: Lasting powers of attorney. This is when a person appoints and gives legal authority to another person to act in his or her best interests in relation to personal, health, social or financial welfare. This other person can be a family member or friend;
- **Sections 24–26**: advanced decisions to refuse treatment. This relates to a person's right to refuse, in advance, any nursing or medical intervention or treatment.

ASSESSING MENTAL CAPACITY

PAUSE FOR THOUGHT 6.3

Marcel arrives, unconscious, in the A&E department where Hanif works. Marcel is, consequently, unable to make any decisions about his nursing and medical care. However, he still needs to be assessed and treated. How would Hanif assess Marcel's mental capacity, Marcel's ability to make decisions and what does he do if Marcel cannot make such decisions?

As Marcel is unable to offer, withhold, or withdraw consent to nursing and medical intervention and treatment when he arrives at the A&E department and it would be very wrong to wait until he regains consciousness and his decision-making ability before offering such care, Hanif would have to act in Marcel's best interests in order to safeguard his life. Consequently, Hanif may well be involved in discussions around assessing Marcel's mental capacity under direct supervision of the senior nurse on duty. Such discussions may include the following: does Marcel have either a permanent or temporary impairment of, or disturbance in, the functioning of the mind or brain? Although unconscious and thus meeting this criterion, is this unconsciousness sufficient to imply that Marcel lacks the capacity to make a particular decision? This is known as the 'two stage test for capacity'.

The answer to this second question can be determined by considering whether, after being given all help and support to make the decision, Marcel cannot do at least one of the following:

1. Understand and absorb basic information relevant to the decision to be made
2. Retain the information long enough to process it
3. Weigh up the advantages and disadvantages against his or her value system
4. Communicate his or her decision.

Although unconscious and thus unable to meet all four of these criteria, Marcel only needs to meet *one* of these four criteria to be considered to lack capacity.

As part of this discussion around capacity, a discussion that has to be ongoing given that Marcel is likely to regain consciousness, the issue of 'best interest' must be highlighted (*see 'Section 4' below*). Again, Hanif, being a student nurse who is on duty at the time, is likely to be part of this discussion but will not lead it as this would be the role of more senior and experienced nursing and medical colleagues. Again, decisions around what is and is not in Marcel's best interest are likely to be as a result of team discussions, with the nurse manager and/or doctor taking the ultimate responsibility for such decisions.

Section 4: Best interests

1. In determining for the purposes of this Act what is in a person's best interests, the person making the determination must not make it merely on the basis of:

   a. the person's age or appearance, or

   b. a condition of his, or an aspect of his behaviour, which might lead others to make unjustified assumptions about what might be in his best interests.

2. The person making the determination must consider all the relevant circumstances and, in particular, take the following steps

3. He must consider:

   a. whether it is likely that the person will at some time have capacity in relation to the matter in question, and

   b. if it appears likely that he will, when that is likely to be.

Section 4: Best interests (cont'd)

4. He must, so far as reasonably practicable, permit and encourage the person to participate, or to improve his ability to participate, as fully as possible in any act done for him and any decision affecting him

5. Where the determination relates to life-sustaining treatment he must not, in considering whether the treatment is in the best interests of the person concerned, be motivated by a desire to bring about his death

6. He must consider, so far as is reasonably ascertainable:

    a. the person's past and present wishes and feelings (and, in particular, any relevant written statement made by him when he had capacity)

    b. the beliefs and values that would be likely to influence his decision if he had capacity, and

    c. the other factors that he would be likely to consider if he were able to do so.

7. He must take into account, if it is practicable and appropriate to consult them, the views of:

    a. anyone named by the person as someone to be consulted on the matter in question or on matters of that kind

    b. anyone engaged in caring for the person or interested in his welfare

    c. any donee of a lasting power of attorney granted by the person, and

    d. any deputy appointed for the person by the court, as to what would be in the person's best interests and, in particular, as to the matters mentioned in subsection (6).

8. In the case of an act done, or a decision made, by a person other than the court, there is sufficient compliance with this section if (having complied with the requirements of subsections (1) to (7)) he reasonably believes that what he does or decides is in the best interests of the person concerned

9. "Life-sustaining treatment" means treatment which in the view of a person providing health care for the person concerned is necessary to sustain life

10. "Relevant circumstances" are those:

    a. of which the person making the determination is aware, and

    b. which it would be reasonable to regard as relevant.

(www.legislation.gov.uk/ukpga/2005/9/section/4)

The basic rule here is to act in the least restrictive way possible under the circumstances. Remember to ensure that any decision made in another person's best interest regarding his or her care follows organisational policies and protocols, is made with the agreement of all stakeholders and is recorded and documented thoroughly.

THE ROLE OF THE NURSE

Whilst this chapter may appear to be overly wordy and legalistic, unfortunately it had to be so as the MCA is, by definition, a legal document. So, let's 'rewind the clock' a bit.

Having been involved in a road traffic accident, Marcel arrives unconscious at A&E where Hanif works as a student nurse. Is Hanif required to seek Marcel's consent prior to providing nursing care?

Because he is unconscious, Marcel is unable to provide, refuse or withdraw consent (**MCA Section 2:1**). Whilst this does not mean that Hanif can ride roughshod over what Marcel would have preferred had he been in a position to give consent, Hanif is permitted to provide emergency life-sustaining nursing care (**Sections 1:3, 4:10**). Hanif would not be guilty of assault as long as he acted in Marcel's best interest, in line with departmental policies and protocols and in good faith. In relation to Marcel's 'best interest', it is vital that all other people engaged in Marcel's care are involved in decision-making (**Sections 4:6a–c, 7a–b**). This must include: other nurses, doctors, Marcel's family and any advance statement that Marcel had written. It is vital that any nursing care (and medical care for that matter) is arrived at through a consensus of professional and family views and opinion and **must be recorded**, along with the reasons for the interventions and the reasons why consent could not be given by Marcel. Marcel's level of consciousness and his ability to decide and consent must be reviewed regularly and acted upon (**Section 4:3a–b**).

Once Marcel has recovered consciousness and his pain and distress levels do not impede his decision-making and consent-giving abilities, then he must be encouraged to participate in nursing intervention decisions and consent (**Section 4:4**).

Because of Marcel's learning disability, Marcel is likely to need information presented to him in simpler ways that he is more likely to understand. Therefore, without being patronising or condescending to Marcel, Hanif should seek the assistance of those who work and live with him and, if possible, the learning disability liaison nurse on how to present information to Marcel in ways that he can understand.

PAUSE FOR THOUGHT 6.4

Marcel has now been transferred to the general medical ward. It is the evening 'drug round' and Marcel refuses his medication. Is it right to try to disguise his medicine by mixing it with his food? Discuss.

In times gone by, it was fairly common practice to administer medicine by mixing it with food. However, Marcel has a right to make decisions, in this case to refuse to give consent to accept his evening medication, for a good reason, a bad reason or for no reason at all and that having a learning disability is not grounds for believing that Marcel is unable to give consent (**Section 2:3b**). Try to find out why Marcel is refusing his medication and work around this. It could be that Marcel does not like the nurse who is administering the medication, that he has friends or family visiting, that he is tired or for many other reasons. If it is possible, in the case of the former, ask a colleague who Marcel likes to administer the medication or come back at a later time to administer the medication. The same applies to any other forms of nursing intervention such as meeting his personal hygiene needs (washing, dressing, toileting, shaving, etc.). As Marcel is likely to be anxious and frightened as a result of having been hit by a car and being in a strange and alien environment, try to enlist the help of his family and the learning disability liaison nurse.

CONCLUSION

Consent and the mental capacity to give, refuse to give or withdraw such consent have been highly complex and thorny legal, philosophical, ethical, nursing and medical issues for decades. This is true not only for those with a learning disability but for many other patient or service user groups such as the elderly, young teenagers and those who experience mental health issues. Despite the existence of the Mental Capacity Act 2005, issues around consent and mental capacity are likely to persist for the foreseeable future. However, Marcel's rights to refuse and withdraw consent need to be respected, promoted and safeguarded in order to provide high-quality care and to avoid any accusation of abuse.

KEY POINTS

- Those with a learning disability have the right to refuse and withdraw consent to treatment and interventions for a good reason, a bad reason or for no reason at all.

- Consent can be expressed or implied.

- For consent to be valid, the following criteria must be met. The consent has to be based on sufficient relevant information, voluntary and given by somebody who is capable of giving consent.

- The stated aims of the Mental Capacity Act 2005 are to provide a statutory framework that will empower and protect vulnerable people who are unable to make their own decisions and to make clear who can take decisions on the behalf of another person and in what circumstances.

- The Mental Capacity Act encompasses such issues as consent, best interest, lasting power of attorney, deprivation of liberty and courts of protection.

REFERENCES

Hobden, A. & Mills, S. (2008) Consent and capacity *in* Clark, L. & Griffiths, P. (2008) *Learning Disability and Other Intellectual Impairments: meeting needs through health services.* Chichester, John Wiley & Sons.

McIver, M. (2006) Legislation and learning disability *in* Peate, I. & Fearns, D. (2006) *Caring for People with Learning Disabilities.* Chichester, John Wiley & Sons.

The Mental Capacity Act 2005 can be downloaded from www.legislation.gov.uk/ukpga/2005/9/introduction

07

LEARNING DISABILITY AND MENTAL HEALTH

AIMS AND LEARNING OUTCOMES:

The aims of this chapter are to:

- Investigate the meaning of mental health from a clinical and service user perspective

- Explore the various forms of mental health problems

- Highlight the prevalence of mental health issues within those with a learning disability

- Explore the various forms of therapeutic intervention that are available when working with those who have a learning disability who also experience mental health issues.

By the end of this chapter you will:

- Have a basic understanding of the meaning of mental health

- Be aware of the various forms of mental ill-health

- Be aware of how many people with a learning disability are also likely to experience mental health problems

- Be aware of how to work with this client or patient group.

INTRODUCTION

Many years ago it was thought, even if anecdotally, that those with a learning disability were unable to develop mental illnesses or mental health problems, as to do so requires a certain level of mental, cognitive and intellectual development, ability and functioning. It was believed that those with a learning disability may not have the intellectual or cognitive level 'needed' to experience mental illness (Smiley, 2005). However, anyone who works with those with a learning disability within a hospital, a residential or a community setting will be very much aware that those with a learning disability can indeed experience the same mental health issues that are prevalent within wider society (Barber, 2011). Again, it could be argued that there is much misunderstanding within society at large, a misunderstanding and even lack of understanding that is reflected in the nursing profession (Priest and Gibbs, 2004) regarding the differences between mental health and learning disabilities, with some people believing that these are the same thing. Maloret (2006) suggests that this lack of understanding may be a result of a lack of education in the area of mental health and learning disabilities.

It is likely that as a staff nurse, a student nurse or a health care assistant working in a general hospital, GP practice, health centre or community nursing team you, the reader, are likely to meet and work with people who have both a learning disability and who are experiencing a mental health problem.

WHAT IS MENTAL HEALTH?

PAUSE FOR THOUGHT 7.1

Mental health, mental illness, psycho, schizo, depressive, nuts, bonkers, mad…. What's in a name?

It must be stated at the outset of this chapter that learning disability is not the same thing as a mental illness or mental health condition. Having a learning disability is not the same thing as having clinical depression, bipolar disorder or schizophrenia, for example.

Sometimes, it is said that a person with a learning disability may have a 'dual diagnosis'. By this is meant having both a learning disability *and* a mental health problem. This can sometimes appear confusing as the term 'dual diagnosis' can also refer to those who experience mental health problems and who use / misuse drugs such as cannabis, cocaine, heroin or alcohol. Those with a learning disability are not immune to such drug use and therefore both senses of the term 'dual diagnosis' can apply. Due to a possible 'overlap' of behavioural signs and symptoms (Maloret, 2006), misdiagnosis of mental health problems within those with a learning disability can sometimes happen, with mental health problems being dismissed as being an aspect of what it is to have a learning disability. So, what is mental health and is mental health the same as mental illness?

It may be helpful here to look at the word 'health'. Health is both an absence of illness and the optimum 'performance' of the body. Therefore mental health could be seen as both an absence of mental illness and the 'optimum performance' of the person's mental and cognitive faculties and mind. However, the World Health Organization defines health as 'being a state of complete physical, mental and social well-being and not merely the absence of disease or infirmity' (www.who.int/about/definition/en/print.html).

Mental illness could be argued to have a number of definitions and meanings.

These include:

A **mental health problem**, as defined by the American Psychiatric Association, is: "a clinically significant behavioural or psychological syndrome or pattern that is associated with present distress or disability or with a significantly increased risk of suffering death, pain, disability or loss of freedom" (APA, 1994). Basically, this means that 'a mental health problem exists when there is a change in a person's behaviour, thought processes or mood to the extent that day-to-day life is adversely effected' (Maloret, 1996).

Mental disorder: Weller (1997: 365) suggests that this term was defined by the Mental Health Act 1983 to cover all forms of mental illness and disability, including mental impairment and psychopathic disorder.

Mental illness: a category not defined by the Mental Health Act 1983 or any other mental health related legislation and which is therefore left open to interpretation. The use of the term 'mental illness' is, however, established through common practice and case law (previous legal cases which have set legal precedents; sometimes referred to as 'judge-made law') as meaning 'the opinion of psychiatrists, backed up by the official classification of mental illness' (Parsons, 2003: 501). However, mental illness could also be described as a term that is used to describe a number of disorders of the mind that affect the emotions, perceptions, reasoning or memory of the individual (Weller, 1997: 365). Parsons (2003) also suggests that mental illness has no definition as such and its meaning is left open to interpretation. Such a position could imply that mental illness is whatever the psychiatrist, psychologist or mental health nurse says it is.

Mental hygiene: 'the science that deals with the development of healthy mental and emotional reactions' (Weller, 1997: 365). This term has also been used in the past to define or categorise mental illness. However, this term could have somewhat negative and unhelpful connotations regarding the moral standing of the person; whether the person who has and experiences a mental health issue is morally and socially 'unhygienic' or 'unclean'.

Again, the use of certain, often negative, language to define a person's mental state could allow the 'non-mentally ill' to exercise control and power over those who experience mental health problems or difficulties.

FORMS OF MENTAL ILL-HEALTH

Having briefly looked at a number of basic, if contrasting and even conflicting, definitions of mental health and mental illness, attention will now be shifted to highlight the various forms that mental ill-health can take. I am indebted to Mark Allen Publishing and the *British Journal of Health Care Assistants* for their kind permission to include the following information from Barber (2011) in this section.

There are wide varieties and forms of mental ill-health which include the following:

Depression: Depression can be seen as 'a morbid and long-lasting sadness or melancholy which may, or may not, be a symptom of an underlying psychiatric problem' (Weller, 1997: 120). Causes of depression are likely to be numerous and symptoms may include:

- Persistent lowered mood for most of the day
- Decreased interest, pleasure or non-engagement in previously enjoyed daily or weekly activities
- Difficulty in sleeping
- Significant weight gain or loss
- Chronic feelings of being worthless, useless and a failure
- Diminished ability to think, concentrate or make decisions
- Thoughts of death, dying, self-harm or suicide.

Bipolar conditions: This used to be known as 'manic depression' and is characterised by a single or multiple episodes of dramatic and severe swings between the two extreme poles of severe mania and severe depression. Bipolar conditions are chronic and recurrent, with the manic phase sometimes requiring hospital admission and treatment.

Dementia: Dementia is a gradual but global and progressive death of brain cells leading to a gradual and irreversible decline in all areas of mental functioning, including memory, intellect, social judgment, personality, social skills/behaviour and physical skills. While dementia is usually associated with old age, it is not unheard of for symptoms to appear at any age.

Addictions: These are a persistent, compulsive dependence on a behaviour (such as sex, work, gambling or shopping) or substance such as alcohol or drugs.

Anxiety disorder: Anxiety is a normal part of what it is to be human; it is a normal aspect of human experiences. Anxiety conditions can be seen as an extreme anxiety response to certain memories, experiences or anticipated experiences and unwarranted worrying can either cause or trigger anxiety states. Physical and behavioural symptoms of anxiety may include:

- Palpitations
- Sweating and dry mouth
- Elevated blood pressure
- Fear, apprehension, sense of impending doom, terror or dread
- Altered sleep patterns
- Irritability
- Panic.

Attention deficit and hyperactivity disorder (ADHD): ADHD is characterised by abnormal levels of inattention, hyperactivity, or their combination. The person must present with the following: inattention (usually has difficulty maintaining attention in activities) and hyperactivity/impulsivity (is often 'on the go' or often acts as if 'driven by a motor').

Obsessive–compulsive disorder (OCD): An obsession is a persistent, often intrusive and unwanted thought, emotion or behaviour that the person cannot ignore. A compulsion is a behavioural manifestation of the obsessive thought. Such behavioural manifestations could include the performance of a repetitious, uncontrollable but seemingly purposeful act or ritual, such as the constant washing of hands, constant checking to see if the lights are turned off or the front door is closed and locked.

Schizophrenia: According to Keen (2003: 258), the diagnosis of schizophrenia refers to a complex and controversial group of conditions. Major symptoms could include:

- Delusional thinking and perceptions
- Auditory hallucinations or 'thought echo'
- Broadcasting, withdrawal or insertion of thoughts into a person's head
- Thought disorder, 'word salad', loosened associations
- Obsessive preoccupation with fantasy and esoteric ideas
- Showing less interest, enthusiasm or emotion than usual
- Inappropriate behaviour.

Borderline personality disorder (BPD): This is a collection of personality traits that underpin certain groups of behaviours including:

- Frantic efforts to avoid real or imagined abandonment
- A pattern of unstable/intense interpersonal relationships
- Markedly and persistently unstable self-image or sense of self
- Potentially self-damaging impulsivity
- Recurrent suicidal behaviour
- Chronic feelings of emptiness
- Inappropriate, intense anger or inability to control anger
- Short-lived stress-related paranoid thoughts.

PREVALENCE

Having briefly looked at the varied forms of mental health issues, problems and conditions that many people can experience throughout their lives, how many people with a learning disability are likely to experience these issues and problems? People with learning disabilities are likely to experience the complete spectrum of mental health problems, with higher prevalence than in those without learning disabilities, as can be seen from *Table 7.1*.

The Foundation for People with Learning Disabilities suggest that "children and young people with learning disabilities are much more likely than others to live in poverty, to

Table 7.1 *Prevalence of mental health conditions in the UK*

Mental health conditions	Those with a learning disability (1–1.5 million)	General UK population (around 60 000 000)
All mental health problems	25–40% (36% of children and adolescents (FPLD, 2012))	25% (8% of children and adolescents (FPLD, 2012))
Schizophrenia	3%	1%
Depression	12.5%	2.8%
Bipolar	1.5%	1–2%
Anxiety disorder	16.7%	8–12%
OCD	2.5–9.4%	1.2%
Dementia	21.6% (those with Down's syndrome are at particularly high risk of developing dementia, with an age of onset 30–40 years younger than the general population)	5.7%
Autism spectrum conditions	Around 35% (FPLD, 2012)	1–1.1%

Sources: Keen (2003) Smiley (2005); Devine *et al.* (2010); Mental Health Foundation (2011a).

have few friends and to have additional long-term health problems and disabilities such as epilepsy and sensory impairments. All these factors are positively associated with mental health problems" (FPLD, 2012).

According to the Foundation for People with Learning Disabilities (2012), 10–15% of people with a learning disability are also likely to exhibit 'challenging behaviours' (aggression, destruction, self-injury and others) with age-specific prevalence peaking between the ages of 20 and 49.

However, caution must be exercised in a number of areas.

Although autism is a condition recognised by the American Psychiatric Association in its 'DSM-IV/5', *it is not a mental health condition in itself*, even if many of those on the autism spectrum are likely to experience mental health issues at a higher level than in the general population. Autism is more a developmental than a mental health condition. Indeed, many people who are on the autism spectrum, particularly those with Asperger's syndrome or high-functioning autism will not experience either a learning disability or a mental health issue and will thus fall between the cracks of service provision.

Whilst 'challenging behaviour' such as aggression, anti-social behaviour and self-harm can often be a sign or symptom of a mental health issue, it is not a mental health condition in itself.

The reader should be aware of, and exercise caution in potentially pathologising normal or near-normal human responses to normal life experiences as mental health issues. One such example is the inclusion of bereavement as a potential mental health condition in '*DSM-5*'.

While anecdotal evidence suggests a link between mental ill-health and learning disabilities, actual prevalence in percentage terms of mental health problems in people with a learning disability can prove to be somewhat elusive. In other words, according to Barber (2011), it is uncertain how many people with a learning disability will also experience a mental health problem. Even Mencap, in response to a personal emailed enquiry from the author, does not hold such data and was thus unaware of prevalence or comparison rates in terms of those without a learning disability.

There are 'lies, damned lies and statistics' (a phrase often attributed to the 19th century British Prime Minister Benjamin Disraeli and popularised by the American writer Mark Twain amongst others)! Beware of misusing or accepting the simple statistics given in this chapter and throughout the book at face value.

THE ROLE OF THE NURSE

> Tariq is a 48-year-old gentleman with Down's syndrome, 'voice hearer' and severe anxiety disorder. Following a minor stroke at the care home where he lives, Tariq has been admitted to the general medical ward where Hanif works as a student. As Hanif has previously indicated an interest in mental health issues, he has been asked to assist in Tariq's care during his stay on the ward.

Although learning disability and mental ill-health are not the same issue, those with a learning disability are statistically more likely to experience a mental health problem than those who do not have a learning disability, and Tariq is no different.

Reading Tariq's notes, Hanif finds that Tariq, although admitted to the hospital ward following a minor stroke, has a number of underlying mental health issues which have no connection to the stroke. According to his notes, Tariq is a 'voice hearer' who also experiences severe anxiety issues. Observing and interacting with Tariq, Hanif comes to believe that he is also experiencing depression. What are Hanif's roles in Tariq's care?

Initially, Hanif's role is to become fully aware of Tariq's mental health history and how the mental health issues impact upon Tariq's daily life. Hanif should be able to do this through a combination of:

- Interacting with, talking with and listening to Tariq
- Reading Tariq's nursing and medical notes

- Talking to those who are significant in Tariq's life such as his family and his support workers
- Seeking the advice of the learning disability liaison nurse and visiting mental health nurse, psychologist and psychiatrist.

Having become aware of Tariq's mental health history and its impact on his life, Hanif could find out what is 'normal' behaviour and mood for Tariq. This may sound strange but be aware that everyone has a slightly different take on what 'normal' is: what is 'normal' in terms of mood and behaviour for one person may not be 'normal' for someone else. Also, what may be a problem in terms of mental health behaviour for one person may not be a problem for another. Hanif should work within that individualised understanding.

Communication will play a vital role in meeting Tariq's holistic needs whilst on the ward. This includes communicating with colleagues, family and, above all, Tariq. It must be remembered that connecting psychologically and emotionally with Tariq through communication and interaction is a basic human need and right and that mental ill-health is not catching! Communicating with Tariq may make it easier and less intrusive to observe for any subtle changes in his mental state, his mood and his behaviour.

There are a number of therapeutic forms that could be helpful to Tariq in managing his mental health problems.

Pharmacotherapy: Drugs such as chlorpromazine and haloperidol (management of psychosis), lithium carbonate (management of bipolar conditions), nitrazepam (night-time sedation), fluoxetine (management of depression) and diazepam and lorazepam (management of anxiety disorders) could be helpful here. These drugs have been used for many decades to manage behavioural and mood disorders in those with a learning disability. It is likely that as Tariq experiences auditory hallucinations and severe anxiety issues, he would already be using medication to manage his symptoms. Hanif's role is to encourage Tariq in continuing his medicine regime whilst he is in hospital, to answer any questions that Tariq may have about his medication and to monitor, report and record any drug benefits and side-effects that Tariq may be experiencing.

Talking therapies: Talking therapies, including cognitive behavioural therapies (CBT), dialectic behaviour therapy (DBT), psychodynamic therapies, humanistic therapies, and support and information, give people the chance to explore their thoughts and feelings and the effect they have on their behaviour and mood. For more on 'talking therapies' for those with mental health problems, please see the Mental Health Foundation website (2011b). Caution must be exercised here as there appears to be a lack of research as to the effectiveness of the variety of available 'talking therapies' on those with a learning disability.

Complementary therapies: These will include hypnotherapy, reiki, meditation, acupressure, acupuncture and prayer or other spiritual exercises. Although used for centuries in China,

India and Japan, their effectiveness with those with a learning disability is under-researched and under-tested and must therefore be used with great caution. However, a wide range of complementary therapies are becoming more popular in the UK and as many of these forms of therapy rely to a large extent on holistic human connectedness and compassion, they can rarely be unsafe.

CONCLUSION

Although learning disability and mental ill-health are not the same phenomenon, people with a learning disability are as likely as, and indeed are perhaps more likely than anyone else to experience mental health problems. Consequently, it is more than likely that, at some point in Hanif's nursing career, he will engage and support those with a dual diagnosis of learning disability and mental health issue. It is thus hoped that this chapter on learning disability and mental health will have aroused your interest in this fascinating area of work.

KEY POINTS

- Those with a learning disability are as likely as, and perhaps more likely to experience mental health issues than anyone else.

- A mental health problem is a clinically significant behavioural or psychological syndrome or pattern that is associated with present distress or disability or with a significantly increased risk of suffering death, pain, disability or loss of freedom.

- Mental health issues could include depression, schizophrenia, bipolar (manic depression), severe anxiety, addictions, obsession/compulsion, dementia, ADHD and borderline personality disorder.

- Forms of therapy could include medication, talking and listening to the patient and an increasing range of complementary therapies.

REFERENCES

American Psychiatric Association (1994) *Diagnostic and Statistical Manual of Mental Disorders (DSM-IV)*. Washington, American Psychiatric Association.

American Psychiatric Association (2013) *Diagnostic and Statistical Manual of Mental Disorders (DSM-5)*. Washington, American Psychiatric Association.

Barber, C. (2011) Supporting mental health issues alongside learning disabilities. *British Journal of Health Care Assistants*, 5:11, 548–52.

Devine, M., Taggart, L. & McLornian, P. (2010) Screening for mental health problems in adults with learning disabilities using the Mini PASADD Interview. *British Journal of Learning Disabilities*, 36(4): 252–8.

Foundation for People with Learning Disabilities (2012) *Learning Disability Statistics: mental health issues.* Available at: www.learningdisabilities.org.uk/help-information/ Learning-Disability-Statistics-/187699/ (last accessed 16 October 2014)

Keen, T. (2003) The person with schizophrenia *in* Barker, P. (ed.) (2003) *Psychiatric and Mental Health Nursing: the craft of caring.* London, Arnold Publishers.

Maloret, P. (2006) Mental health issues and adults with learning disabilities *in* Peate, I. & Fearns, D. (2006) *Caring for People with Learning Disabilities.* Chichester, John Wiley.

Mental Health Foundation (2011a) *Mental Health in People with Learning Disabilities.* Available at: www.mentalhealth.org.uk/our-news/blog/1102-06-23/ (last accessed 16 October 2014)

Mental Health Foundation (2011b) *Talking Therapies.* Available at: www.mentalhealth.org. uk/help-information/mental-health-a-z/T/talking-therapies/ (last accessed 16 October 2014)

Parsons, S. (2003) Psychiatric Legislation: an international perspective *in* Barker, P. (ed.) *Psychiatric and Mental Health Nursing: the craft of caring.* London, Arnold Publishers.

Priest, H. & Gibbs, M. (2004) *Mental Health Care for People with Learning Disabilities.* London, Churchill Livingstone.

Smiley, E. (2005) Epidemiology of mental health problems in adults with learning disability: an update. *Advances in Psychiatric Treatment*, 11: 214–22.

Weller, B. (1997) *Baillière's Nurses' Dictionary.* 22nd edn. London, Baillière Tindall Ltd.

08

LEARNING DISABILITY AND FORENSIC CARE

AIMS AND LEARNING OUTCOMES:

The aims of this chapter are to:

- Briefly discuss the meaning of forensic services and care

- Tentatively present the numbers of those with a learning disability who are likely to come into contact with forensic services as either victims, perpetrators or witnesses to crime

- Chart a number of potential journeys through forensic services

- Present a number of ways in which those who encounter forensic services can be supported.

By the end of this chapter you will:

- Be able to discuss what forensic services and care involve

- Have an understanding of how many people with a learning disability are likely to come into contact with the forensic services

- Have accompanied three people with a learning disability in their journey through forensic services and care

- Be able to discuss a number of ways that those who come into contact with forensic services can be supported.

Victoria, a 20-year-old woman with a mild learning disability, has been arrested by the police for possessing a small amount of a 'Class B' substance (cannabis). This was not the first time that Victoria had come to the attention of the police. Previous encounters had been as a result of Victoria's 'antisocial behaviour' where she received a police caution. This is the first time that Victoria has been arrested for drug-related offences. Victoria lives with her parents who are finding it increasingly difficult to manage her behaviour.

Brian, a 40-year-old with autism and a mild learning disability, has been arrested for sending sexually explicit video images of himself and written material over the internet (using a social networking site) to a 14-year-old girl. This offence was compounded by asking the girl to masturbate while watching the video images that he had sent her. Brian lives on his own but with multi-agency support. This was Brian's first offence.

Yasmin, a 30-year-old with mild learning disability and autism who lives with her parents, has been subjected, on the grounds of her disability, to verbal and physical violence for the past three years by groups of youths and their parents who live on the same housing estate as she does. Yasmin arrives at her local police station after being kicked and punched by these youths.

INTRODUCTION

It could be suggested that a person with a learning disability is probably as likely as any other person to come into contact with the various branches of the criminal justice system and with forensic services, either as a victim of crime, a witness to crime or a perpetrator of a crime (Barber, 2011). When discussing the proposal for this book with a colleague, the issue of whether or not to include a chapter on forensic care was raised. A number of nurses, nursing students and health care assistants are likely to be working within the criminal justice and forensic care services or even in more generic community services, who may well come into contact and work with crime victims or perpetrators who have a learning disability. Therefore, it would be appropriate for this chapter to be included here.

WHAT ARE FORENSIC SERVICES?

There are three forms of forensic services. The first is the solving of crimes through scientific investigations. If one watches TV programmes such as the British 'Silent Witness' or the American 'Body of Proof', for example, one may already be aware of this aspect of forensic services. The second is the criminal justice system which includes the police, the courts and the probation services. Forensic services also means a sub-branch of psychiatry that serves as the interface between the law, the various aspects of the criminal justice system such as the courts, prisons and the probation service and psychiatry and residential or community mental health services (Burrow, 1993). This chapter will focus on the second and third aspects of the term 'forensic services'.

Kingdon (2009: 361) suggested that although there have been forensic services of sorts as far back as 1863, there is no nationally agreed definition of forensic services or the roles of those who work with them. Indeed, most, if not all, of the 19th and early 20th century psychiatric institutions would have been what today would be called 'secure environments' and could thus be seen as 'forensic' in nature. Furthermore, an acceptable and universal definition of forensics and therefore what comprises forensic services is elusive (Kettles *et al.*, 2001; Baxter, 2002). However, Chaloner and Coffey (2000) did suggest that "Forensic nursing is about the assessment, treatment and management of mentally disordered offenders across a spectrum of secure environments, including the community".

Put somewhat simply, the type of behaviour that would lead a person to access forensic services is any behaviour that would bring the individual into contact with the various arms of the criminal justice system, mainly the police, the courts and custodial services. This could include: arson, theft, burglary, physical assault, drug possession and supply, sexual assault (including rape), 'hate / mate crimes', kidnapping and 'conduct likely to cause a breach of the peace' such as fighting in public or rioting. In all of these crime areas, the person with a learning disability can be a victim, a witness or a perpetrator.

In the context of forensics, learning disability is considered as a mental disorder and those with a learning disability as mentally disordered (United Kingdom Central Council for Nurses and University of Central Lancashire, 1999; Kearns, 2001). Kingdon (2009: 366) suggests that people who come to the attention of the forensic services are likely to be those who have a borderline to mild learning disability.

The term 'forensic services' could be broken down into the following services, all of which staff nurses, student nurses or health care assistants could potentially work in or come into contact with.

Prisons: Here, nurses will meet the physical and mental health care needs of prison inmates, regardless of whether the inmate has been previously diagnosed with a learning disability or mental health issue. For information on prison nursing see the Royal College of Nursing's (RCN) Nursing in Criminal Justice Services Forum or its Forensic Nursing Forum (see *References and Resources*).

Secure settings: Again, nurses within secure settings, such as Rampton Hospital in Nottinghamshire, will meet the physical, mental and emotional needs of the service users within a holistic framework. Services at Rampton, for example, will include mental health, female services, learning disabilities and personality (including dangerous and severe) disorders.

Medium to low community-based secure settings: Medium security settings are those that provide a residential and therapeutic environment and service for those convicted of a crime but who present a serious but less immediate danger to others and have the potential to abscond. Low security settings are intended for those patients who present a less serious physical danger to others. Their security measures are intended to impede rather than prevent absconding, with greater reliance on staffing arrangements and less reliance on physical security measures.

Forensic psychiatry: This is a service that provides a bridge between mental health services and the criminal justice services.

PREVALENCE

It appears that large numbers of those who appear before the courts, both young people and adults, are likely to have a learning disability (Jacobson and Talbot, 2009). Whilst it is not known exactly how many people with a learning disability are likely to come into contact with the forensic services either as victims, witnesses or perpetrators of crime, the following statistics should be kept in mind:

- Between 20 and 30% of offenders at any one time have a learning difficulty or learning disability (Jacobson and Talbot, 2009: 5). The Prison Reform Trust (Talbot, 2012) puts this figure somewhat lower, at between 10 and 20%
- Over 60% of children who offend have communication difficulties and, of this group, around half have poor or very poor communication skills (Talbot, 2012)
- Around a quarter of children who offend have an IQ of less than 70 (Talbot, 2012)
- 7% of adult prisoners have an IQ of less than 70 and a further 25% have an IQ of 70–79 (Talbot, 2012)
- Almost 6000 men, women and children with an IQ of less than 70 (those who have a learning disability) are incarcerated in UK prisons at any given time (Reading and Spelling Channel, 2013)
- Prison inmates who have a learning disability are vulnerable to threats to their physical and psychological wellbeing and are more likely to be subject to control and restraint techniques (Allen, 2013)
- People with a disability are significantly more likely to be victims of crime than those without a disability. This gap is largest amongst those aged 16–34, where 39% of people with a disability reported having been a victim of crime, compared to 28% of people without a disability (HM Government, 2014)
- People with a disability are less likely than their non-disabled peers to think the Criminal Justice System (CJS) is fair. This gap is largest amongst those aged 16–34, where 54% of people with a disability think that the CJS is fair, compared to 66% of people who do not have a disability (HM Government, 2014)
- Those who are victims of hate crimes continue to be failed by the police, with many police officers neither properly investigating disability hate crimes nor treating victims as credible witnesses, according to a report by Mencap (*The Guardian*, 20th June 2011).

A JOURNEY THROUGH FORENSIC SERVICES

The journeys through the criminal justice service for Yasmin, Victoria and Brian (the three people we very briefly met at the start of this chapter) are likely to be long and complex. Given the diversity of the issues that surround them, their respective journeys are likely to be very different. Their stories are highlighted below. In the cases of Victoria and Brian, the pathways given in Kingdon (2009, p. 377 (Appendix 12:1)) have been followed. There appear to be no similar pathways for victims or witnesses of crimes.

Yasmin

Yasmin is different from Brian and Victoria as she is a victim of crime rather than its perpetrator. Whilst there is an increasing amount of literature around forensic services and *perpetrators* of crime, there appears to be very little in the way of researched evidence and information on forensic services and *victims* of crime. This apparent lack of research, information and resultant lack of support services for victims of crime is likely to be compounded by police officers not being able to recognise when a victim (and perpetrator for that matter) has a learning disability (Halstead, 1996). The ability to read, write and hold a conversation may mask the real level of disability and whilst the police may be good at recognising moderate or severe learning disability, those with a borderline or mild learning disability may be missed and their needs neither recognised nor met.

How Yasmin is approached by the desk officer at the police station could have either a positive or negative effect on her. As the bullying, victimisation and aggression that Yasmin and her family have experienced have occurred over a three-year period it is unlikely that this is the first time that the assistance of the local police has been sought. Trust or distrust of the police and legal system balances on such assistance and experiences.

It is likely that Yasmin will be asked if she would like to be taken to the local A&E department to have any physical injuries assessed and treated. It would be good practice for Yasmin to be offered the services of an 'appropriate adult' or advocate who could accompany her to the hospital. Once she feels able to do so, a statement of what happened would be taken and the perpetrators, if identified, brought to the police station for questioning. If the perpetrators are themselves children or minors (under the age of 18) then they may be vulnerable in their own right and may need access to similar 'appropriate adult'/advocacy services. Yasmin should be offered ongoing access to 'victim support' services as a matter of course. Victim Support, whilst being neither a government agency or part of the police, is a national charity that gives free and confidential help to victims of crime, witnesses, their family, friends and anyone else affected across England and Wales. Victim Support also speaks out as a national voice for victims and witnesses and campaigns for change (www.victimsupport.org.uk/).

Victoria

After being arrested, Victoria was taken to her local police station where she was assessed by the forensic medical examiner and then interviewed in the presence of an 'appropriate adult' (the local police station will likely have a list of people who could act as an 'appropriate adult'). At the interview, the role of the 'appropriate adult' is to protect the rights of vulnerable adults and children/minors within what is likely to be a highly stressful and often frightening environment and to ensure that those being arrested and interviewed are treated fairly and humanely. After the interviewing officer sought advice regarding the most appropriate way to deal with Victoria, and given that this is not the first time that Victoria had been in contact with the police due to her behaviour, she was charged with possession of a Class B drug rather than just cautioned. Victoria was released on bail before being ordered to appear before the magistrates' court. Throughout the entire process, Victoria was supported by both the forensic and community learning disability nursing teams to understand why she had been arrested, what her rights were, the legal processes, what was happening to her at the police station and what was likely to happen to her over the next few weeks prior to and after appearing at the magistrates' court. Given that this is not the first time that Victoria had come to the attention of the local police due to her behaviour, it was felt that a police caution would not be effective or appropriate at this time.

The magistrate, having again sought advice from appropriate support agencies, based his decision on the fact that Victoria does have a learning disability and that a custodial sentence would not provide any real benefit for Victoria or society. The magistrate decides instead to sentence Victoria to a non-custodial community service along with ongoing input regarding her use of drugs and antisocial behaviour. To this end, Victoria is offered support and guidance by the forensic learning disability and mental health teams.

Brian

Brian was arrested at his home address as a result of a formal complaint being made by the victim and her parents. Brian was taken to the local police station where he was assessed by a forensic medical examiner (often a local GP who is contracted to provide medical services such as assessments on people who have been arrested) and then cautioned and interviewed in the presence of an 'appropriate adult'. Although the nature of the offence was serious, it was decided that to release Brian on police bail prior to appearing before the magistrates' court was the appropriate action to take. However, due to the nature of the offence, it was felt that to issue Brian with a police caution would not be appropriate.

Although Brian apologised for his behaviour and promised that it would never happen again, because of the severity of the offence and the age of the victim (being under the age of consent), the magistrate invoked Section 35 of the Mental Health Act 1983 which permits for the hospital detention of a person for assessment. During his time within a community-based low secure unit, Brian was further assessed and supported to understand why he had acted as he did and to realise that his behaviour was wrong. He was also made aware of the effects and consequences of his actions on himself and others, including the possibility and effects of being placed on the 'sex offenders register'. After a period within the low secure unit, Brian was reassessed and, as it was considered that he no longer posed a threat to society, released with ongoing support and supervision by the community forensic and learning disability teams.

THE ROLE OF THE NURSE

We have already met Jill and Hanif from the introductory chapter. Jill is a health care assistant who works in a GP practice and Hanif is a student nurse (adult branch) who is now completing a short assignment in a local police station as part of his learning disability placement. What are their roles in meeting the holistic needs of Brian, Victoria and Yasmin?

Brian and Victoria

Hanif may well participate in the following:

- Observing and offering appropriate and supervised assistance in the physical, emotional and psychological assessment of Brian and Victoria
- Engaging in conversations with Brian and Victoria. This will, in part, gain their trust and could form part of the holistic assessment process
- Acting as an 'appropriate adult' if asked to do so during police interviews
- Advocating on behalf of Brian and Victoria whilst they are in custody
- Accompanying Brian and Victoria to the magistrates' court for moral support. It is unlikely that Hanif will have the necessary skills and knowledge to act as an 'expert witness' on behalf of either Brian or Victoria, this being the role of the forensic nursing team
- Visiting and supporting Brian in the low secure unit and Victoria during her community service, and observing and participating in any rehabilitation programmes that Brian and Victoria will undergo.

Jill, the HCA, may be involved in the ongoing support through the provision of health checks of Brian and Victoria once they have been released or discharged back into the community. Jill may also be involved in the finding and securing of appropriate overnight or weekend respite care for Victoria so that her parents can have a break. Again, Jill may become involved in facilitating support groups not only for Victoria's parents and any siblings but for other parents and siblings in a similar position. Finally, Jill may be involved in supporting Victoria's parents to obtain carers' benefit, carers' grants and access to local authority, NHS or voluntary sector run carers' support services.

Yasmin

Here, Hanif's role is likely to include:

- Observing and offering appropriate assistance in the physical, emotional and psychological assessment of Yasmin
- Engaging in conversations with Yasmin to gain her trust
- Acting as an 'appropriate adult' and advocate during police interviews, and
- Accompanying Yasmin to the local A&E so that she could have her injuries assessed and treated.

Again, as a placement project, Hanif could investigate the existence and effect of hate crimes against those with a learning disability within the community and of discrimination against those with disabilities within the health care systems (RCN Congress, 2013).

It would be inappropriate for either Hanif or Jill to offer 'quick fix' approaches to long-standing disability hate crime such as that experienced by Yasmin and her family. Even the police appear to downplay the existence and effects of hate crimes on people with a learning disability and their families (*The Guardian*, 20th June 2011). It would certainly be inappropriate to suggest that Yasmin and her family move to a different area of town or a different town entirely, although on the surface such a move may result in a cessation of the hate crimes that they have experienced. Having said that, both Hanif and Jill could be aware of and involved in the Mencap campaign on hate crime (see Mencap's 'Stand by me' campaign: www.mencap.org.uk/campaigns/take-action/stand-me).

CONCLUSION

As can be seen, those with a learning disability are just as likely to come into contact with the various aspects of forensic services, either as perpetrators, witnesses or victims of crime. These services and the issues and behaviour that are connected to forensic services tend to be complex and do not lend themselves to simple 'quick fix' solutions. Nonetheless, the roles of the forensic psychiatric team can be fascinating and rewarding areas to investigate further and to work in, as can the prison health services. Indeed, some health care assistants, nursing students and newly registered nurses may already be working in these fields. Riding *et al.,* (2005) may prove to be a useful resource for those who are, or are considering such a role.

KEY POINTS

- Those with a learning disability are as likely as anyone else to come into contact with forensic services, as either a witness, victim or perpetrator of a crime.

- Forensic services include the criminal justice system and a sub-branch of psychiatry that serves as the interface between the law, the various aspects of the criminal justice system and psychiatry and residential or community mental health services.

- The role of the nurse, nursing student or health care assistant will include reassuring the service user, offering psychological, emotional and practical support and acting as an 'appropriate adult' and advocate.

REFERENCES AND RESOURCES

Allen, D. (2013) The other side of the bars. *RCN Bulletin* (September 2013).

Barber, C. (2011) Support for learning disabilities in forensic services. *British Journal of Health Care Assistants*, 5:10; 491–494.

Baxter, V. (2002) Nurses' perception of their role and skills in a medium secure unit. *Mental Health Nursing*, 11:30; 1312–1319.

Burrow, S. (1993) An outline of the forensic nursing role. *British Journal of Nursing*, 2:18; 21–38.

Chaloner, C. & Coffey, M. (eds) (2000) *Forensic Mental Health Nursing: current approaches*. Oxford, Blackwell Sciences.

Halstead, S. (1996) Forensic psychiatry for people with a learning disability. *Advances in Psychiatric Treatment*, 2: 76–85.

HM Government (2014) Disability facts and figures. Available at: http://odi.dwp.gov.uk/disability-statistics-and-research/disability-facts-and-figures.php#js (last accessed 11 November 2014)

Jacobson, J. & Talbot, J. (2009) *Vulnerable Defendants in the Criminal Courts: a review of provision for adults and children*. London, The Prison Reform Trust.

Kearns, A. (2001) Forensic services and people with learning disability: in the shadow of the Reed Report. *Journal of Forensic Psychiatry*, 12:1; 8–12.

Kettles, A., Peternelj-Taylor, C., Woods, P. *et al.* (2001) Forensic nursing: a global perspective. *British Journal of Forensic Practice*, 3:2; 29–41.

Kingdon, A. (2009) Forensic learning disability practice *in* Jukes, M. (ed.) (2009) *Learning Disability Nursing Practice*. London, Quay Books.

Reading and Spelling Channel (2013) Crime and Reading Problems. Available at www.readingandspellingchannel.com/crime-and-learning-disabilities.html (last accessed 11 November 2014)

Riding, T., Swann, C. & Swann, B. (eds) (2005) *The Handbook of Forensic Learning Disabilities*. Oxford, Radcliffe.

Royal College of Nursing (RCN) Congress (2013) 22. Disability discrimination. Available at: www.rcn.org.uk/newsevents/congress/2013/agenda/22-disability-discrimination) (last accessed 11 November 2014)

Royal College of Nursing's (RCN) Forensic Nursing forum: http://www.rcn.org.uk/development/nursing_communities/rcn_forums/forensic

Royal College of Nursing's (RCN) Nursing in Criminal Justice Services Forum: www.rcn. org.uk/development/communities/rcn_forum_communities/prison_nurses

Talbot, J. (2012) *Fair Access to Justice? Support for vulnerable defendants in the criminal courts.* London, Prison Reform Trust.

The Guardian (2011) *Police are Failing People with Learning Disabilities, Says Study.* Available at: www.theguardian.com/society/2011/jun/20/police-failing-learning-disabilities-study (last accessed 16 October 2014)

United Kingdom Central Council for Nursing, Midwifery and Health Visiting and University of Central Lancashire (1999) *Nursing in Secure Environments.* London, UKCC.

09

SEXUALITY AND PEOPLE WITH A LEARNING DISABILITY

AIMS AND LEARNING OUTCOMES:

The aims of this chapter are to:

- Highlight the meaning of sexuality

- Briefly highlight a variety of issues around sexuality and those with a learning disability

- Briefly discuss the law relating to sexual relationships and those with a learning disability

- Briefly discuss issues around consent to sexual activity

- Highlight the roles of the nurse in relation to the sexuality of those with a learning disability.

By the end of this chapter, you will be aware of and understand:

- The meaning of sexuality and sex

- How the various aspects of human sexuality impact upon those with a learning disability

- The law and sexuality

- Issues around consent and sex

- Your role as a staff nurse, a student nurse or a health care assistant in promoting appropriate sexual health.

INTRODUCTION

Human sexuality, along with dying, death and bereavement, is perhaps one of the most difficult aspects of working with those who have a learning disability that nurses, nursing students or health care assistants are likely to encounter. After all, personal politics, sex and dying/death/bereavement are still very much socially taboo subjects; one does not talk about them in public. They are the rather large 'elephants in the room'; they exist but few people even acknowledge them, let alone discuss them! Most people will just dance around the issues that are raised by human sexuality, often employing euphemisms in order to hide embarrassment. This could also apply to nurses. Therefore, within 'polite society', human sexuality and learning disability are likely to make for a very odd couple indeed!

However, to deny that those with a learning disability are sexual beings, that they have a right to their sexuality and that they have a right to experience and express their sexuality on the same basis as anyone else, is a gross denial of their human dignity, their human rights and of what, in part, makes them human.

WHAT IS SEXUALITY?

Those with a learning disability are sexual beings, the same as me and you and they have the same need and drive to sexually define, experience and express themselves as such. However, what is sexuality?

Sexuality could mean different things to different people at different times and in different cultures, with issues around self-identity, image, sensuality and sex being perhaps some of the more common and important concepts. Human sexuality focuses on a wide array of attributes and social activities and an abundance of behaviours, series of actions and societal attitudes. Again, sexuality can be seen as the quality or state of being sexual. Quite often, sexuality is an aspect of one's need for closeness, caring, and touch. Generally speaking, human sexuality is how people experience and express themselves as sexual beings. Human sexuality also involves the capacity to have erotic experiences and responses. Human sexuality may also involve a person's sexual attraction to another person which may be determined by their sexual orientation (gay, lesbian, bisexual or heterosexual ('straight')). Human sexuality impacts upon cultural, political, legal and philosophical aspects of life. It can refer to issues of morality, ethics, theology, spirituality or religion.

Within a wide variety of societies, sexuality can be defined, in part, by an increasing number of cultural contexts and governed by implied rules and social norms. Even within a single society (such as 'British', 'French', 'German' or 'Italian'), there are a number of often distinct and competing sub-cultures. By this it is meant that language, history and popular culture have roles to play in defining and promoting sexuality. One has only to see how colour mediates gender and sexuality in babies and very young children: even now, many baby girls are dressed in pink and baby boys in blue. As one gets older, more and more aspects of contemporary life and culture help to define, shape, present and express sexuality. Clothing colour, toys, play and social activities, music, TV programmes, films, sports, advertising and cosmetics are all examples of the culture of sexuality. However, as these are likely to be social and historical constructs, i.e. sexual meanings and norms that are 'artificially constructed' by society, such as the rise of feminism and the sexual revolution (Foucault, 1976), the experience and expression of sexuality can and quite often do change over time. Here time is seen in terms of decades and centuries on one level and over the course of an individual's life span on another.

The age and manner in which children are informed of issues of sexuality are often hotly debated and are usually seen as a matter for parents and school-based sex education to resolve. Different countries hold varying views on when (ranging from age-appropriate pre-school to puberty and teenage years) and how such sex education is presented, the contents of such education programmes and who teaches or presents these programmes. However, even within a single country, there has often been much discussion and conflict as to the nature of sex education programmes and many 'faith-based' schools unwillingly accepting the need for such programmes, often placing 'sex education' within a wider context of a loving and caring relationship.

ISSUES REGARDING SEXUALITY AND THOSE WITH A LEARNING DISABILITY

PAUSE FOR THOUGHT 9.1

Imagine if your sexuality was denied or deemed to be wrong just because it exists. Hormones are not aware that they are seen by some as 'inappropriate' just because the bodies they inhabit are disabled. (Clark, 2014)

Sexuality is likely to encompass a wide range of relationships, behaviours and issues. This is true for everybody, whether they have a learning disability or not. Some of these issues will include many of the following:

- Gender issues: the complex interplay of historical and current social and cultural influences and expectations that help to shape a person's sexual identity
- Puberty: a developmental and maturation stage which marks the start of the transition between childhood and adulthood that everyone experiences, whether or not they have a learning disability. Wrobel (2003) provides a wealth of useful information that could be invaluable when supporting pre-teenagers or teenagers with a learning disability and their parents
- Masturbation: if done in private, this is a normal means of sexual release
- Sexual relationships
- Contraception
- Marriage
- Pregnancy, either within or outside marriage
- Same-sex relationships

- Alternative forms of sexual expression such as receiving and giving physical pain for sexual pleasure, bondage and fetish wear and pornography (both 'straight' and 'gay/lesbian').

Those with a learning disability are people first and learning disabled second. Thus, those with a learning disability have the same rights and drives as anyone else to engage in sexual activities and having a learning disability must not preclude engagement in such activities. Sexually transmitted conditions such as genital herpes, gonorrhoea and chlamydia may be seen by some within society almost as a 'badge of honour' and an acceptable consequence of a free sexual expression and experience. However, those with a learning disability also have a right to protection from these infections and advice **must** be sought from the multi-disciplinary team if it is believed that a person or couple with a learning disability is sexually active and at risk of contracting a sexually transmitted infection.

People with profound and multiple learning disabilities (PMLD), such as Thomas (from previous chapters) are likely to have the same needs and rights to explore their bodies, to derive pleasure from doing so and to express and experience their sexuality, as anyone else. However, as a result of the profound level of their learning disability they would be unable to validly give, withhold or withdraw voluntary consent to any form of sexual relationship. Therefore, it would be illegal for anyone to engage in a sexual relationship with those with a PMLD. Having said that, the sexuality of those with a PMLD, as for other people with a learning disability, can be asserted through the use of clothing fashions, hair styles, cosmetics, room décor and 'gender-biased' music styles and social activities. For more information, see Mencap (2008).

However, those with a learning disability can be both victims and perpetrators of sexual abuse. Sexual abuse or abusive relationships occur when consent to such sexual or emotional/'romantic' relationships or activities was not freely given by either party. This could involve a range of behaviour ranging from unwanted sexual attention, 'nuisance' phone calls, 'sexting' (the sending of text messages with a sexual content) and stalking to sexual assault and rape. Forced marriages and female genital mutilation, both prevalent in certain cultures, are also forms of sexual abuse. Again, the administration of oral contraception without the person's knowledge or consent and the administration of certain hormones to either slow down or prevent the onset of puberty (particularly in females) can be seen to be abusive. In previous generations both of these occurred. Some of these issues and behaviours could arise from a lack of knowledge, awareness and understanding of what comprises appropriate sexual behaviour and could be addressed through education.

THE LAW

Those with a learning disability are both subject to and protected by the same legislation that every other person is subject to and protected by. Within the UK, no-one under the age of 16 can consent legally to sex regardless of ability, although this age of consent may differ in other countries, and sex with a child under 12 years of age is considered to be statutory rape. According to the Sexual Offences Act 2003 it is an offence to engage in 'sexual activity with a person with a mental disorder impeding choice'. A person with a serious or profound learning disability, by the nature of this definition, is unlikely to have the capacity to consent to sexual activity, (i.e. to understand what it means and its possible consequences). This means they are likely to fall into the category of a person who has a 'mental disorder impeding choice'. However, does, and should, this apply to the same degree to those with a borderline or mild learning disability, given that such people are likely to be more aware of choices and their consequences and thus more likely to be able to consent?

It is also an offence to:

- Cause or incite a person with a mental disorder impeding choice to engage in sexual activity
- Engage in sexual activity in the presence of a person with a mental disorder impeding choice
- Cause a person with a mental disorder impeding choice to watch a sexual act.

Although intended to act as safeguards for those who are likely to be vulnerable to sexual abuse and exploitation because of their learning disability, the problem here is that this could potentially become a 'blanket ban' on all 'legitimate' sexual expression, experience and activity on the part of those with a learning disability. Therefore, great care must be taken to ensure that those with a learning disability are protected from sexual, physical, mental and emotional harm through sexual exploitation whilst acknowledging that they are sexual beings and have the same right as anyone else to express and experience their sexuality. For more information see Mencap (2008).

ISSUES AROUND CONSENT

It could be suggested that consent and the ability to give consent is the central key issue that needs to be considered in relation to sex and people with a learning disability. It must be remembered here that any sexual act such as intimate touching or kissing without consent is sexual assault and that having sex with a person without that person's consent is rape. It must also be remembered that consent to kissing or the holding of hands is not the same as, nor does it imply, consent to the person having sex. This applies to everyone, regardless of whether or not that person has a learning disability.

In England and Wales, the relevant legislation is in the Sexual Offences Act 2003 and the Mental Capacity Act 2005 (Thompson, 2011). For people aged 16 and over, section 74 of the Sexual Offences Act says: "A person consents if he or she agrees by choice and has the freedom and capacity to make that choice". Without such consent, an offence has been committed. It is also illegal for staff and volunteers to have sex with the people they support and care for (Thompson, 2011).

The Mental Capacity Act 2005 formed the central component of *Chapter 6*, where the meanings of mental capacity and consent and how to assess a person's ability or mental capacity to give a valid consent were discussed. Put simply, consent, which could either be explicit or implicit and verbal, written or gestural, refers to the provision of approval or agreement between two or more people or between a person and an organisation, particularly and especially after thoughtful consideration, for an action to take place. For the purposes of section 2 of the Act, a person is unable to make a decision for himself if he is unable to: understand the information relevant to the decision, retain that information, use or weigh that information as part of the process of making the decision and communicate his decision (whether by talking, using sign language or any other means).

There are a number of principles within the Mental Capacity Act 2005 that may be relevant to assessing whether a person with a learning disability has the necessary mental capacity to consent to a sexual relationship. These include:

- Assume capacity: many people with learning disabilities are likely to have the mental capacity to engage in sex and relationships
- Support people to make their own decisions: provide appropriate and accessible information on relationships, healthy living and sex education
- People can make unwise choices: a bad relationship is a mistake we can all make
- If someone lacks capacity the decision must be in their best interests: assess capacity to consent to sex
- Try to limit restrictions on the person's rights and freedom: where an individual lacks capacity to consent to sex it may not always be in his or her best interests to stop opportunities for sexual contact.

In order for consent to be valid, those with a learning disability should understand what sex involves physically and emotionally, and that it should feel good. They should also understand the potential consequences of sex, such as pregnancy, sexually transmitted infections (STIs) and the risk of emotional hurt, as well as the importance of consent for both parties involved, including the right to say no (Thompson, 2011). However, Thompson (2011) also suggests that the most difficult capacity assessments involve people with learning disabilities who agree to have sex but may lack insight into the other person's motives. Examples may include the woman with a learning disability agreeing to have sex on the promise of a relationship, but not understanding that the man is only interested in sex, or a man with a learning disability thinking he has a girlfriend, but she is mainly interested in his benefits or having somewhere free to stay. In either of these scenarios, the person with a learning disability may be the victim of a crime under the Sexual Offences Act 2003.

It is likely that there may be a number of people with a learning disability who are gay, lesbian or bisexual. However, those who are face enormous challenges to 'come out' as such, and it may be some time before significant numbers are able to make this choice for themselves (Abbott and Howarth, 2005; Clark, 2014).

It should be borne in mind that mental capacity assessments can be subjective, and two different care professionals may come to different conclusions about the same case. If a consensus cannot be achieved, it may be necessary to ask the Court of Protection to decide on a person's mental capacity to consent to engaging in a sexual relationship.

THE ROLE OF THE NURSE

Jill (briefly introduced in *Chapter 1*) is a health care assistant who works in a GP practice three days a week and a local community health centre for the remaining two days. In both settings, she works with a number of people ranging from 15 to 70 years of age who have a learning disability. Jill is interested in providing effective support to her patients/service users in the area of sexual health.

Human sexuality involves many complex emotional, ethical, social, moral and legal issues. Therefore, for Jill to offer responses to questions or queries, that may seem to be simplistic in nature, from those with learning disabilities, is likely to be unhelpful, inappropriate and bordering on the unprofessional. However, there are a number of things that Jill can do in order to provide an effective support service.

- Although she is a health care assistant and not a registered nurse and as such is not (yet) subject to the professional code of conduct for nurses, it would be good practice for Jill to be aware of, understand and work within the Nursing and Midwifery Council's (NMC) code of professional conduct. She must never forget that she is personally and professionally accountable for her actions (or lack of them)
- Jill needs to be aware of, understand and implement fully any employer and organisational procedures, policies and guidelines around the issues of sexuality, sexual health and consent
- Jill needs to be aware of and understand that she does not work in a social, ethical, philosophical or cultural vacuum. Therefore, she must be aware of and understand how these issues impact upon what she does and how she does it
- Jill must actively listen in a compassionate and non-judgmental manner that takes into account both what the service users are saying and what they are not saying
- Jill could ensure that accurate and up-to-date information regarding a wide range of sexual issues such as puberty, contraception, STIs, straight/same-sex relationships, pregnancy/childbirth and parenthood are made available in a variety of formats including videos/DVDs, easy read and visual (line drawings, pictures and photos)

- There are a number of resources that Jill could access for advice and support in order to assist her service users. These could include hospital-based learning disability liaison nurses, the local learning disability services or mainstream sexual health care or health promotion professionals. Jill could also seek the advice of the sexuality support team where such teams exist (see box below) before implementing any sexual health programmes. Although this particular service is rare and the one cited below is based in Hertfordshire, the team highlighted below have a national as well as a regional remit. Thus it may be useful to contact them for advice and suggestions. Any sexual health programmes must be drawn up using a multi-disciplinary team approach.
- Jill could set up and sensitively facilitate workshops on healthy living and lifestyles and parenting (Brickley, 2003; Woodhouse *et al.*, 2001). Such workshops could include many of the issues covered briefly in the sections above. To avoid the problems that could arise through a perception on the part of service users that Jill is 'preaching' a healthy lifestyle message, such workshop sessions must be run by those with a learning disability and be guided by their wants, needs, and agenda.

What is a Sexuality Support Team?

The Sexuality Support Team is an initiative run by the Hertfordshire Partnership University NHS Foundation Trust.

The Sexuality Support Team (SST, formerly *Consent*) offers a range of services to respond to a broad range of sexuality issues affecting women and men with learning disabilities, including enabling informed choices, sexual health, issues of HIV risks, and working with people with learning disabilities who have been sexually abused or perpetrated sexual abuse.

The team has a multi-disciplinary approach and has a national profile for quality and experience. The SST is part of Hertfordshire Partnership NHS Trust, but offers its services across the UK and aims to work in partnership with other individuals and organisations.

Services include consultancy, group work, training, individual work, workshops, conferences and student placements. Other NHS Trusts may operate something similar to this. It may also be useful to contact the SST at Hertfordshire Partnership University NHS Foundation Trust either for information regarding similar teams in other parts of the UK or ideas on how to set up and run your own teams.

Tel: 01923 670796

Web: www.hertspartsft.nhs.uk/working-for-us/training-anddevelopment/consent/

CONCLUSION

As those with a learning disability develop and grow older, their sexuality is a fact of life which needs to be faced, accepted and engaged with. Those who work with people who have a learning disability walk a very thin tightrope when it comes to that person's sexuality. On the one hand, nurses, nursing students and HCAs have a professional and common-law duty of care and protection to those who have a learning disability (just as they have to any other vulnerable patient or service user). On the other hand, those with a learning disability have a basic human right to experience, express and enjoy their sexuality on the same basis as anyone else. This right must be remembered and acted upon appropriately at all times.

KEY POINTS

- Those with a learning disability have the same sexual needs, desires and drives as anyone else in society.

- Sexuality means different things to different people at different times and in different cultures, with issues around self-identity, image, sensuality and sex being perhaps some of the more common and important concepts.

- Sexuality can be asserted through the use of clothing fashions, hair styles, cosmetics, room décor and 'gender-biased' music styles and social activities.

- The Sexual Offences Act 2003 put in place a range of measures to safeguard those with a learning disability from sexual abuse.

- Consent and the ability to give consent is the central issue that needs to be considered in relation to sex and people with a learning disability.

REFERENCES AND RESOURCES

Abbott, D. & Howarth, J. (2005) *Secret Loves, Hidden Lives: issues for gay, lesbian and bisexual people with learning difficulties*. Bristol: Norah Fry Research Centre.

Brickley, S. (2003) Working with parents who have a learning disability and their children *in* Jukes, M. & Bollard, M. (eds) (2003) *Contemporary Learning Disability Practice*. Salisbury, Mark Allen Publishing.

Clark, N. (2014) Let's talk about sex. *Enable* (July/August 2014), pp. 33–34.

Foucault, M. (1976) *The History of Sexuality Vol. 1: an introduction*. Paris, Editions Gallimard.

Mencap (2008) Sexuality and people with profound and multiple learning disabilities (PMLD)? Available at: https://www.mencap.org.uk/sites/default/files/documents/2008-04/Mencap_Sexuality_and_people_with_PMLD.pdf (last accessed 14 November 2014)

Mencap (2011) A Court of Protection decision about sterilising a woman with a learning disability has been adjourned until May. 15 February 2011. Available at: https://www.mencap.org.uk/news/article/court-protection-decision-about-sterilising-woman-learning-disability-has-been-adjourne (last accessed 14 November 2014)

Nursing Times (2011) Decisions about sex for people with learning difficulties. Available at: www.nursingtimes.net/nursing-practice/clinical-zones/learning-disability/decisions-about-sex-for-people-with-learning-disabilities/5033828.article (last accessed 11 November 2014)

Thompson, D. (2011) Decisions about sex for people with learning disabilities. *Nursing Times*, 107: online edition, 23 August.

Woodhouse, A., Green, G. & Davies, S. (2001) Parents with learning disabilities: service audit and development. *British Journal of Learning Disabilities*, 29: 128–132.

Wrobel, M. (2003) *Taking Care of Myself: A hygiene, puberty and personal curriculum for young people with autism*. Arlington (Texas), Future Horizons.

10

AGEING AND THOSE WITH A LEARNING DISABILITY

AIMS AND LEARNING OUTCOMES:

The aims of this chapter are to:

- Discuss the meaning of old age
- Highlight normal ageing
- Highlight a number of medical, physiological, neurological and sensory issues associated with the ageing process
- Highlight issues around dementia
- Briefly highlight the role of the nurse.

By the end of this chapter, you will be aware of, understand and be able to discuss:

- The meaning of old age
- What constitutes 'normal ageing'
- The impact of a number of medical issues associated with ageing
- The impact of dementia on those with a learning disability
- Existing services and the need for both generic and specific services for those with a learning disability
- Your role as a nurse, a nursing student or an HCA.

SCENARIO 10.1

Jim, a 67-year-old gentleman with a severe learning disability, is experiencing the early stages of Alzheimer's dementia. Jim lives in a residential home for those with a learning disability along with four other people, where the average age of the residents is 60 and the youngest resident is 50.

INTRODUCTION

Life expectancy for those with a learning disability has been slowly increasing since the 1920s to the point where many of those with a learning disability are now expected to live into what would normally be seen as 'old age' (Ouldred & Bryant, 2008; Yang *et al.*, 2000; Mencap, 2013). However, it has only been fairly recently that any serious thought has been given to the possibility that those with a learning disability may reach and live well into old age. Consequently, whilst services and resources for those who are elderly and do not have a learning disability exist and are usually excellent, the existence of both generic and specific care and support services for people who have a learning disability as they enter and live through old age may range from non-existent to excellent via poor, patchy and good.

It is likely that as a staff nurse, a student nurse or a health care assistant (HCA) working in a general hospital, GP practice, health centre, community nursing team or elderly residential care services you are likely to meet and work with people with a learning disability who are experiencing old age.

WHAT IS OLD AGE?

PAUSE FOR THOUGHT 10.1

When does old age occur? Does one actually know when one reaches old age? Does it matter?

The inclusion of the two poems ('*Warning*' and '*Radio 2*') referred to below, although light-hearted, is intended to question attitudes related to ageing and what is considered to be 'appropriate old age related behaviour'.

PAUSE FOR THOUGHT 10.2

Humorous poems on ageing

Is ageing and old age a state of mind? Before reading the remainder of this chapter, read the two humorous poems on ageing (the first of these two may be familiar to many of you):

- '*Warning*' by Jenny Joseph (available at www.poemhunter.com/poem/warning/) (about a woman's rebellion against ageing)

- '*Radio 2*' by Dean Farnell (available at: www.dennydavis.net/poemfiles/aging2b.htm).

For some of us, old age is so far away that it does not even register; for others, it is just around the corner beckoning to us! Yet, do we actually know what old age is and when middle age ends and old age starts? Is a basic meaning of old age applicable to everyone?

It could be suggested that old age is very much a 'moveable feast', with those who have reached the retirement age of 66 considering themselves or being considered to be moving into old age. Yet, many people who are in their 70s and beyond still consider themselves to be 'middle-aged' or youthful, at least in spirit! One has only to look at the main characters in the television sitcom '*Last of the Summer Wine*' that can still be viewed on Youtube and certain digital TV channels! Is there a mismatch between what a person's body is telling them and what their mind and soul are telling them? This debate is pertinent when one considers that many people who are in their 70s are still working for a living, some (such as a number of major religious leaders) in very high profile and very demanding roles. One has only to look at Pope Francis, who was 76 when he took office in March 2013!

Again, those with a learning disability are known to have a life expectancy below that of those without a learning disability. However, they also tend to experience many of the health issues that are associated with old age, such as dementia, well before their 'non-disabled' peers.

For the sake of expediency, the current retirement age of 66 will be taken as marking the end of middle age and the start of old age. However, as the age of retirement is set to rise, so should the start of 'old age'.

NORMAL AGEING

As can be seen from the two poems cited above, ageing can be rather bittersweet, with a gradual rather than abrupt onset. Physical appearance may change: grey hair to be replaced by white hair and smooth skin by wrinkles. Many will remember with clarity and perhaps with some sadness their youth and may try to deny their advancing years. I, for example, will fully intend to enter my 70s and 80s still listening to and enjoying Pink Floyd, Gong and Genesis (the Peter Gabriel years of course)! There are likely to be grandchildren and even great-grandchildren to enjoy and embarrass. The mortgage will be paid off and there may be more money and time for leisure activities such as the University of the Third Age (U3A), travel, gardening, and arts and crafts. Meeting friends for tea, coffee or the odd pint or two may become more important as methods of social engagement. The need for personal reflection on one's life, the need for reconciliation with friends and family members and personal religious faith, beliefs and activity may become more important during the ageing process.

More negative aspects of normal ageing include the realisation of one's own mortality and having a finite time left to live. More and more of one's friends and family will die (although only 55 years old, I am aware of around half a dozen people from my own year at secondary school who have died). The body may start to show major signs of 'wear and tear' and consequently many people who are elderly may need greater assistance with normal activities of daily living. There may be more social isolation, loneliness and consequent depression.

COMMON MEDICAL CONDITIONS

Although those with a learning disability who are elderly are at vastly increased risk of developing dementia, there are a wide range of health and physical conditions which they are also at increased risk of developing. However, these may not be recognised as such, because nurses may feel that these conditions are part of the person's learning disability rather than the effects of ageing. These health and social conditions are likely to include some or many of the following.

Visual impairment. Ouldred and Bryant (2008) suggest that visual impairment, up to and including becoming registered blind, is likely to increase with age and level of disability and may even be higher in those with a learning disability. This is particularly marked in those with Down's syndrome (Wallace and Dalton, 2006). It appears that the most frequent form of visual impairment in those with a learning disability is cataracts, with a prevalence rate of around 40% in people with Down's syndrome.

Hearing impairment. As with visual impairment, hearing impairment also increases with age and again is more common in those with learning disabilities, particularly Down's syndrome (Wallace and Dalton, 2006).

Depression. Many elderly people are likely to experience depression for a variety of reasons, including social isolation, loneliness, the death of family and friends, the person's own impending death and increasing physical and sensory frailties.

Hypothyroidism. Hypothyroidism can occur in 20–30% of people with Down's syndrome (Ouldred and Bryant, 2008) and means that the thyroid gland does not produce enough hormones. Common signs of an underactive thyroid, some of which can mimic certain signs and symptoms of dementia, are tiredness, weight gain, functional decline and feeling depressed. An underactive thyroid is not usually serious and can often be treated successfully by taking daily hormone replacement tablets such as thyroxine.

Coronary artery disease. This is a disease of the arteries which supply blood to the heart and is the second most common cause of death amongst those with a learning disability; it is increasing as a result of the rise in life expectancy and lifestyle changes (Ouldred and Bryant, 2008). Up to 50% of those with Down's syndrome have some form of congenital heart defect which exposes those with such defects to increased risk of strokes and heart attacks.

Epilepsy. Drugs used to manage and treat epilepsy may cause drowsiness and problems with physical co-ordination and movement, both of which may be confused with dementia symptoms.

Diabetes. Although the prevalence of both type 1 and 2 diabetes in people with learning disabilities is unknown, it is generally thought (Ouldred and Bryant, 2008) that both types are more common than in those without a learning disability. Complications associated with diabetes, including retinopathy, neuropathy and nephropathy, are likely to increase with age.

Arthritis and other musculoskeletal conditions. These are conditions that affect people increasingly as they get older and which negatively affect their physical mobility and dexterity, with pain becoming increasingly difficult to manage. This is true for both those with and without a learning disability, although the onset of arthritis in those with a learning disability could well be earlier. Thus meeting their own personal hygiene needs, opening items such as bottles, cans or jars, using ordinary cutlery and getting out of the house become increasingly difficult.

Social isolation. Social isolation is *not* inevitable as a result of advancing age and its accompanying physical and health issues. However, as a result of increasing sensory, memory, physical and mobility difficulties, increasing numbers of elderly people appear to lose confidence in going out independently. This may result in a gradual decline in social contact and interaction and the loss of friends, some of whom may also be experiencing social isolation for similar reasons. Those with a learning disability may already experience such social isolation as a result of their existing disabilities and may thus feel any increased isolation more keenly.

DEMENTIA

Ouldred and Bryant (2008, p. 89) suggest that "as people with pre-existing intellectual impairment grow older they become subject to developing the same health conditions and problems as the older general population". They also suggest that the prevalence of dementia is much higher in those with a learning disability and that many health and social care professionals are unaware of, or do not understand the increased risk of Alzheimer's dementia or its symptoms in people with learning disabilities. Indeed, Prasher (1995) suggests that dementia, the most prevalent form of which is Alzheimer's disease, can be present in around 36% of those with a learning disability who are aged 50–59. Although deterioration in other human faculties such as mobility, sight and hearing can normally be seen within an elderly population, it is perhaps dementia that is most commonly identified with old age. This is also particularly true for those with a learning disability.

What is dementia? Ouldred and Bryant (2008, p. 90) suggest that dementia is a syndrome that affects memory, thinking, orientation, comprehension, calculation, learning capacity, language and judgement. Alzheimer's disease is characterised by a build-up of abnormal proteins between nerve cells and a reduction of chemical neurotransmitters such as acetylcholine. There is a gradual progression of the disease, starting from the area of the brain that controls and regulates memory and which will eventually affect all areas of the brain.

Assessment of dementia

Early diagnosis of dementia conditions in people with a learning disability is likely to be complex. However, it is vital in order that conditions such as depression and thyroid problems, which may mimic some of the symptoms of dementia, can be treated and then ruled out. According to Ouldred and Bryant (2008), the best place to carry out a diagnostic assessment for dementia is in the person's own home, as this is likely to be the most familiar and non-threatening environment for the person.

There have been a number of studies into the diagnosis of dementia conditions in people with a learning disability. For example, DC–LD, the classification system developed by the Royal College of Psychiatrists (2001) is one of the tools that are often used to diagnose dementia, and Aylward *et al.,* (1997) have published international guidelines on the diagnostic criteria for the diagnosis of dementia conditions in people with a learning disability.

When assessing adults with a learning disability such as Jim (see *Scenario 10.1*) in order to diagnose possible dementia, the following may be useful:

- Jim's physical appearance and the appearance of his immediate environment
- Perceptions
- Jim's mood: does he appear depressed?
- Thought process
- Insight: is Jim aware of what is happening to him?
- Does Jim express and experience compulsive and repetitive rituals?
- Has Jim's personality changed?
- Is Jim oriented to person, time, place, memory or language? Does Jim know who and where he is and what day of the week, month of the year or year it is?

Much of the evidence for the above can be gained through spending time and interacting with Jim and observing him around the home where he lives. The home's care staff, other care professionals and Jim's care, nursing and medical notes will also be a valuable source of information. Such sources of information become even more important if Jim does not have or loses the ability to communicate verbally.

THE ROLE OF THE NURSE

With advancing old age of those with a learning disability and its accompanying mental, sensory and physical frailty and possible isolation, the roles of the nurse are likely to be many, varied and challenging.

First of all, there is a need to understand the ageing process and its associated health conditions, such as dementia, and how this process can affect the person. This could be achieved through engaging in professional development opportunities such as workshops, short courses and the reading of journal articles around the ageing process and care for the elderly.

Secondly, try to resist the temptation of approaching and treating all those with a learning disability who are elderly together as one group. They are individuals first and foremost and then elderly learning disabled; they deserve and have the right to be treated accordingly! Having said that, there are a number of things which those working with people who have a learning disability and are elderly could find useful, including:

- *Verbal and gestural reassurance* being given to those such as Jim who are experiencing age-related health conditions.
- *Accurate and current information* regarding the various health care issues being experienced by Jim must be made available to him in a format and manner, and at a time appropriate to his needs, levels of understanding and ways of communicating.
- *Pharmaceutical management* of some of the symptoms of dementia. Don't forget that there is no known cure for dementia. However, cholinesterase inhibitors appear to be effective in the symptomatic slowing down and relief of cognitive decline (Ouldred and Bryant, 2008).
- *Reality orientation and validation*, which aims to maintain and improve the person's orientation and awareness of their environment through a variety of prompts and activities (Ouldred and Bryant, 2008). Validation therapy focuses on the importance of an individual's feelings and their attempts to express them instead of correcting factual errors in communications. The true meanings behind the communication are sought.
- *Reminiscence therapy* seeks to encourage recollections and memories of details or events of an individual's life. Reminiscence therapy, which can take place either one-to-one or in a small group setting, can have a positive effect on a person's autobiographical memory, socialisation, long-term memory, communication and social interaction and engagement.
- Some, like Jim, will live in a local authority, health service or independent sector care home. The care home staff may need support in meeting Jim's holistic care needs.

The provision of domiciliary care and support for those who live on their own with multi-agency support could be invaluable not only in the meeting of physical needs such as dressing/undressing, nutrition/hydration, mobility and personal hygiene but in social communication, interaction and engagement. Don't forget that one of the major issues that many elderly people have to face on a daily basis is social isolation.

Likewise, specialist daily living equipment should be provided, such as magnifying glasses (to enable those with declining eyesight to read printed material such as letters, books and newspapers), bottle and can openers, raised toilet seats, large-handled cutlery and mobility aids such as walking frames. These can be obtained through the 'Nottingham Rehabilitation' catalogue, the local physiotherapy team, local disability equipment stockists (check the telephone directories or online for details of these) or disability trade exhibitions such as Naidex (see their website: www.naidex.co.uk).

The support, information and resources that can be provided by the various voluntary organisations for those who are elderly should not be overlooked. Age UK, for example, has a very informative website that covers many of the issues experienced by those who are elderly (www.ageuk.org.uk). Age UK also runs local support groups, drop-in centres for those who are 'informal care givers' and outreach services.

Whilst there are a great many suitable and appropriate services for those who are elderly, there may well be a lack of similarly appropriate services for those who have a learning disability and who are elderly. This is particularly likely to be the case when working with those who have a profound and multiple learning disability (PMLD). Therefore, it may be useful to work with the local community learning disability team to design and create appropriate services that meet the holistic care and support needs of people like Jim or those with a PMLD, rather than trying to 'shoehorn' them into existing services that are too generic to meet their needs.

CONCLUSION

This chapter has sought to highlight some of the health and care support needs of those who, like Jim, have a learning disability and age-related health conditions such as dementia. Some of these needs are likely to be very similar to those of any other elderly person, whilst others may be unique to those with a learning disability, particularly those with PMLD. The emphasis of nursing care and support must be to enable those who are elderly to enjoy their remaining years. Rather than having *'One foot in the grave'*, those with a learning disability should be able to enjoy being the *'Last of the summer wine'*.

KEY POINTS

- Life expectancy of those with a learning disability is changing significantly, with increasing numbers reaching and living well into old age.

- Old age does not necessarily have to involve decreasing physical and mental health, with increasing numbers of very active people who are in their 70s and 80s.

- Those with a learning disability who do live into old age are likely to experience similar social and health issues as other elderly people including sensory impairment, mobility problems, heart conditions, depression, arthritis and social isolation.

- Dementia is likely to be a major health and social issue as around a third of all those with a learning disability are expected to develop dementia.

- The role of the nurse, nursing student and HCA is likely to be very challenging as the possibility that those who have a learning disability reaching old age has only recently been planned and provided for.

REFERENCES

Aylward, E., Butt, D., Thorpe, L. & Dalton, A. (1997) Diagnosis of dementia in individuals with intellectual disability. *Journal of Intellectual Disability Research*, 41: 152–64.

Mencap (2013) *Health: later years.* Available at: www.mencap.org.uk/all-about-learning-disability/health/later-years (last accessed 16 October 2014)

Ouldred, E. & Bryant, C. (2008) The older adult: intellectual impairment and the dementias *in* Clark, L. & Griffiths, P. (2008) *Learning Disability and Other Intellectual Impairments.* Chichester, John Wiley & Sons.

Prasher, V. (1995) Age-specific prevalence, thyroid dysfunction and depressive symptomology in adults with Down syndrome and dementia. *International Geriatric Psychiatry*, 10: 25–31.

Royal College of Psychiatrists (2001) *DC–LD: diagnostic criteria for psychiatric disorders for use with adults with learning disabilities / mental retardation.* Gaskell, RCP.

Wallace, R. & Dalton, A. (2006) Clinicians' guide to physical health problems of older adults with Down syndrome. *Journal on Developmental Disabilities*, 12:1 Down syndrome (supplement 1).

Yang, Q., Rasmussen, S. & Friedman, J. (2000) Mortality associated with Down syndrome in the USA from 1983 to1997: a population-based study. *Lancet*, 359: 1019–1025.

11

DYING, DEATH AND BEREAVEMENT AND PEOPLE WITH A LEARNING DISABILITY

AIMS AND LEARNING OUTCOMES:

The aims of this chapter are to highlight aspects of:

- Dying

- Death, and

- Bereavement

as they apply to those with a learning disability.

By the end of this chapter, you will be able to discuss the various meanings of, and processes and rituals around:

- Dying

- Death, including the possible death of dreams, hopes and aspirations as a result of having a child with a learning disability

- Bereavement

- The roles of the nurse whilst supporting those with a learning disability and their families.

SCENARIO 11.1

Paul is a 55-year-old gentleman with a moderate learning disability who lives on his own but with support from a multi-agency team. His mother had died some ten years earlier and his 85-year-old father, with whom he is in regular and close contact, has been diagnosed with end-stage renal cancer and has been given only weeks to live. Paul has an older sister, Stephanie, with whom he is also in close and frequent contact.

INTRODUCTION

As with many issues such as politics, religion and human sexuality, dying, death and bereavement are hardly talked about in public and when they are, they are often couched in terms of misguided fear or misguided humour. However, it has been said that there are only three certainties in life: birth, taxation and death! Following on naturally from *Chapter 10*, which focused on elderly care and people with a learning disability, this chapter will focus on dying, death and bereavement.

Dying, death and bereavement are personal issues and experiences that, at some point in our lives, we will all have to acknowledge and face, either as nurses or as ordinary people. Indeed, it is very likely that we will all have to face up to and acknowledge the death of our parents and grandparents. For some, it is the death of a sibling or a child that they have to face. Some people have to face the issues of dying, death and bereavement a lot sooner than others, whilst others do not encounter dying and death until they are themselves middle-aged or even elderly. Those with a learning disability are no different. They, too, will have to face and accept dying, death and bereavement and sometimes face these alone.

DYING

Dying is a complex phenomenon as it encompasses a number of different issues:

- Dying as the end of life that is usually associated with old age
- Dying as a gradual process that could last from minutes to hours, days, weeks, months and even years
- Dying as a personal and even solitary experience
- Dying as a community experience
- Dying as journey to death
- The conflict between this journey and its inevitable conclusion and the fact that the person undertaking this journey is still very much alive.

Dying is also likely to involve a number of different people and sets of relationships that could include:

- Parents watching and being involved in the dying process of their child who has a learning disability
- Parents who are, themselves, dying and are concerned as to how their disabled child would be able to cope with seeing his or her parent dying and what would happen to that child once the parent is dead
- Siblings and partners who are dying
- The person with a learning disability who is dying and who is concerned for his or her parent, sibling, partner or child

- The person with a learning disability who is aware that his or her parent, partner or sibling is dying. Those with a learning disability, according to Wiseman *et al.* (2008), are more likely to be still living with their ageing parents and are thus more likely to witness, experience and be part of this dying process.

All of these relationships, dynamics and situations are different and will require different approaches in engaging, communicating and working with those who are involved in this dying process.

End of life care, be it for the parent as in *Scenario 11.1*, the sibling, the partner or the person who has a learning disability, is likely to be a major concern and is likely to involve a number of separate issues.

Where is end of life care to be delivered? Is end of life care to be delivered at hospital, in a care / nursing home, in a hospice or at the patient's own home (hospice at home)? These are very real issues which can have a major impact on Paul, his sister and their father. Indeed, is it appropriate to offer end of life care? End of life care is usually associated with cancer care or dementia; what if the patient does not have cancer or dementia? What if the patient is just dying of old age? Is a service that is geared up to meet the needs of those with various cancers needed or appropriate here?

Issues around appropriate pain relief and management are likely to surface and become increasingly important at this time (Wiseman *et al.*, 2008). Those with a learning disability must be offered the same opportunity as everyone else to manage their pain levels through the use of medication. Just because a person has a learning disability does not mean that they do not feel pain in the same way as anyone else! However, medication, its effects and side-effects must be closely monitored in order to prevent under- or overdosing errors.

Likewise, just because someone is dying does not mean that they are not still living. Therefore, opportunities for engaging in valued social and family activities should be offered but not forced upon the person.

Opportunities for the psychological and emotional preparation for the impending death of either the self or the family member must be offered with great sensitivity. Along with this must go the possibility of a need for personal reconciliation either with the self or with others.

Many of those with a learning disability may hold and practice particular religious, cultural or spiritual beliefs. It may be appropriate to seek the support of the person's faith community and its leaders. This is particularly important when one realises that dying and death could be seen as forms of 'rites of passage' with their own religious, spiritual, cultural and community rituals. Such religious and spiritual beliefs and practices may well provide peace and acceptance within the person and thus must never be ignored or ridiculed. Consequently, those with a learning disability should be encouraged, if they so wish, to participate in religious services, rituals and liturgies, preferably at their usual place of worship should they be able to do so.

By so doing, they participate in the ordinary life of their chosen faith community and their faith community has the opportunity to participate in and celebrate the life of one of their members. (See *Chapter 14* for more on spirituality and religion).

DEATH

As with dying, death can be far from simple and can include a range of complex issues.

First, what is meant by death and when does death actually occur? According to Weller and Wells (1990, p. 132) death "is the cessation of all physical and chemical processes that occurs in all living organisms". *Clinical death* is the absence of a heartbeat, determined by a lack of a pulse and the cessation of breathing. *Brain death* is when there is no detectable brain stem activity as manifested by absolute unresponsiveness to all stimuli, absence of all spontaneous muscle activity, and two isoelectric electroencephalograms (the second test being 30 minutes after the first), all in the absence of hypothermia or intoxication by central nervous system depressants. The test for brain death is carried out by two different doctors and the time of death is that time when the second test has been carried out and the patient meets the criteria for brain death.

One of the problems with this basic definition of death is the status of a person, who although to all intents and purposes would meet the criteria for being dead, is nonetheless 'kept alive' through artificial means such as being on a respirator. Is this person dead or alive? This is no mere philosophical or rhetorical question, however, as it arguably underpins the ongoing debate around the therapeutic management of those in persistent vegetative states.

There are likely to be a variety of social, religious, spiritual or cultural rituals surrounding the death of a person. If death occurs in a hospital, it may be useful to contact the relevant hospital chaplain for advice and guidance for some of these rituals. For example, a person with a learning disability who is a Catholic might wish to receive the last rites of the church (what used to be called 'extreme unction') before death occurs. If the person is able, he or she may wish to receive Holy Communion (viaticum) from a priest. Other religions and faith communities may have specific 'rites of passage' immediately prior to and after death.

If the death occurs in a hospital or care/nursing home, be it the death of a person who had a learning disability or his or her parent or family member, the last offices need to be carried out in accordance with local policies and practice. These are the 'last duties' carried out on the body of the deceased by the nurse:

- To prepare the deceased for the mortuary whilst respecting their cultural beliefs
- To comply with legislation, in particular where the death of a patient requires the involvement of a Coroner
- To minimise any risk of cross-infection to any relative, health care worker or other persons who may need to handle the deceased.

Following the death of Paul's father, a number of duties would need to be carried out. These are likely to include:

- Notifying other family members of the death
- Arranging the funeral
- The reading and execution of any last will and testament
- Notifying the Department for Work and Pensions and other relevant welfare benefits agencies so that any welfare benefits and/or pensions that the person received before his or her death be stopped
- Notifying any banks or building societies regarding any bank accounts that the deceased may have held
- Notifying any credit/debit card issuer regarding the cancellation of any cards that the deceased may have held
- Although Paul lives semi-independently, other people with a learning disability may live with their parents. If it is the parent who has died, the accommodation/residential needs of the person with a learning disability who may have been living with him or her may need to be met as a matter of urgency.

Given Paul's learning disability, it is likely that his sister, Stephanie, will have the responsibility for working through these generic duties. Therefore, any nurse or nursing student working with Paul would not be directly involved in carrying out these duties. Indeed, it may well be inappropriate for a nurse to do so. However, the multi-disciplinary team, including nurses, may need to assist Paul to be involved in some of these duties, even if such involvement was limited to being informed of these duties, consulted about how they are to be carried out and knowing that his sister will be directly involved in this process. Paul will also need to be kept informed regarding the progress of these duties in a manner that best meets his emotional and communication needs at the time. Such involvement is likely to form a vital part of the bereavement process and Paul must not be excluded from this process simply because he has a learning disability.

During the days and weeks immediately after the death of a partner, a parent, a sibling or a child, most people are likely to 'operate on autopilot'; most people will therefore need time and assistance to 'work through' the above duties, whether or not they have a learning disability.

BEREAVEMENT

Given that this chapter has tended to focus on end of life issues with dying and death as their inevitable conclusion, either of the person with a learning disability or his or her parent or sibling, bereavement may not be as simple as it may at first appear.

Imagine that you are a new parent who has just received the news that your child (be it born or yet to be born) has Down's syndrome. It is not unusual, even today, for such parents to mourn, to grieve for the child that they will not have and, along with that child, all the hopes, dreams and aspirations that parents would normally hold for such a child. This is a very real form of bereavement and those so bereaved may need extra practical, emotional and psychological support to come to terms with the diagnosis. So, what is bereavement?

Bereavement is a process or journey by which one person mourns or grieves for the loss, usually through death, of another person and which can begin sometimes before the actual death (anticipatory grief) (Hopkins, 2003) and which can last for many years. This other person can be a family member, a friend or sometimes a well-known figure or personality where both the individual and the wider community collectively mourn or grieve for their death. An example of this is the national mourning for Diana, Princess of Wales or Sir Winston Churchill at and after their respective funerals.

Stages of bereavement or grief are likely to include:

- Shock or disbelief, mood swings, loss of concentration, sadness
- Denial of the death or its effects on the person grieving
- Anger at the loss of the person, either through death or through the diagnosis of disability. This anger can be directed either inwardly towards the self or outwardly towards either other people such as health care professionals or the deceased, or at God (however one perceives Him or Her)
- Bargaining
- Depression
- Growing awareness, leading finally to
- Acceptance and hope.

Parker (1996) suggested two further additions: searching, either where the bereaved may have a sense of the dead person still being with them or a searching for meaning and gaining a new identity (taking on roles previously carried out by the dead person in practical matters, personal mannerisms, characteristics and interests).

Grieving may not follow a straight path nor begin at the death of the person. Anticipatory grieving and bereavement may begin prior to death (Hopkins 2003) and may allow time for adjustment to that death to be made (Costello, 1999). Some people miss out on some of these stages whilst others are likely to repeat stages already journeyed through. This journey broadly follows the model of bereavement formulated by Kübler-Ross (1969).

Someone with a learning disability such as Paul may well grieve in the same way as anyone else when they lose someone they love, whilst others will grieve in different ways. Sadly, they may also face more loss than other people, especially if they have friends with a learning disability whose life expectancy may be lower than average (Pearce, 2006). Signs of grief can be difficult to spot, and will be different for each person; some people may get angry, while others may become withdrawn or even destructive. Grief and bereavement can be complicated by:

- The nature of the relationship that the bereaved had with the deceased
- Whether the death was sudden, unexpected or untimely
- Circumstances where many bereavements may have happened together or in quick succession, such as may occur in a serious road traffic or rail accident
- How the deaths occurred
- When a death re-evokes an insufficiently mourned previous death, as may be the case with Paul now that both his parents are dead
- Where there is no family or social support network.

As Paul journeys through bereavement his behaviour may change as a result of being unable to express his feelings verbally (Mencap, 2010; Pearce, 2006). Such changes may include:

- Clinging
- Reluctance to leave the house
- Uncharacteristic incontinence
- Self-injury
- Restlessness
- Aches and pains (often muscular or abdominal)
- Changes in sleep pattern alongside not wanting to sleep on his own
- Changes in or loss of appetite
- Apathy or tiredness
- Minor illness
- Clumsiness and accidents.

Pearce (2006) suggests that those with a learning disability have often been given fewer opportunities to find out about death and bereavement and so may take longer to journey through and resolve their grief over the death of a family member or friend.

THE ROLE OF THE NURSE

Jill works part time in a GP practice and part time in a community health centre as a health care assistant within a community health team. Jill has been asked to work with and support not only Paul but also his sister Stephanie during the period before and after their father's death.

The roles of the nurse when supporting those with a learning disability who are journeying through dying, death and bereavement can be very challenging yet fulfilling.

First, Jill would be well advised to contact the community learning disability team for advice and assistance in providing appropriate support to Paul and his sister during the periods before and after the death of their father. Jill will need to understand that Paul's emotional and psychological needs are likely to be different to those of his sister Stephanie.

Paul and Stephanie must be allowed and helped to prepare for the death of their father in their own ways. This is their right and this right must never be taken away from them. Historically, those with a learning disability were often not informed of the death of their parent or sibling until some time after the death had occurred, and occasionally not even then. The person with a learning disability did not have the chance to say 'goodbye', to be involved in social and religious rituals around dying and death, to attend the funeral or to visit the cemetery. This has often impacted negatively upon the person's behaviour, behaviour that was then wrongly managed.

Jill will need to explain to Paul in simple and honest language what is happening to his father, in terms of the dying and death processes; she must not use euphemisms around dying and death, such as referring to death as 'falling asleep', as a 'loss' or saying that the deceased is now in heaven. This may suggest that those who are dead can be re-awakened or that those who are asleep may be dead. Paul may thus be afraid to sleep at night. 'Death as loss' may suggest that whatever has been lost can be found. Paul may come to believe that the cemetery where his father is buried is in, or is itself heaven. Jill should explain that death happens to everyone and it is when the body has stopped working and cannot be mended. Jill also needs to explain to Paul that his dead father can no longer feel any pain.

Paul should be allowed to view the body of his father if he wishes but must not be forced to do so. He must be allowed to participate alongside his sister in arranging his father's funeral if he wishes. Jill should explain what happens at a funeral and burial or cremation and the roles that Paul may like to take. Paul must be encouraged to talk about his father and listened to with care and compassion. Paul may wish to talk to someone from outside his family and immediate circle of friends and may need support to enable this. A drama, music or art group may be useful in enabling Paul to come to terms with the death of his father and express his grief.

Likewise, designing with Paul a small and simple memorial garden, garden of memories or planting of a memorial tree both as an activity and as a simple ceremony involving Paul's sister and friends could be encouraged. Paul should be assisted to maintain his relationship and contact with his sister Stephanie and other members of his family.

As this aspect of nursing work is likely to be emotionally and mentally draining, Jill must be offered appropriate professional support through supervision and ongoing training and development.

CONCLUSION

The death of a loved family member or friend can often be a very painful and sad experience for anyone, particularly so if they have a learning disability. Yet it can also be a time of great challenge, peace, self-discovery and growth for the individual and those around them. Either way, dying, death and bereavement are not journeys that a person should embark upon alone. After all, this is a journey that all of us, regardless of who we are, will have to take at some point in our lives.

KEY POINTS

- Dying, death and bereavement are normal life experiences that we all have to engage with, either as nurses or as people.

- Dying is a journey to death whilst the person is still very much alive.

- Death is 'the cessation of all physical and chemical processes that occurs in all living organisms'.

- Bereavement is a process or journey by which one person mourns or grieves for the loss, usually through death, of another person and which can begin sometimes before the actual death (anticipatory grief).

- The person with a learning disability is likely to need emotional, psychological and practical support in order to engage with these journeys appropriately.

REFERENCES

Costello, J. (1999) Anticipatory grief: coping with the impending death of a partner. *International Journal of Palliative Nursing*, 5:5; 223–231.

Hopkins, C. (2003) Bereavement and grief counselling *in* Barker, P. (2003) *Psychiatric and Mental Health Nursing: the craft of caring*. London, Arnold.

Kübler-Ross, E. (1969) *On death and dying*. London, Routledge.

Mencap (2010) *Bereavement*. Available at: https://www.mencap.org.uk/sites/default/files/documents/Bereavement.pdf (last accessed 16 November 2014)

Parker, C. (1996) *Bereavement: studies of grief in adult life (3rd edition)*. Harmondsworth, Penguin.

Pearce, J. (2006) *Factsheet: loss, bereavement and death*. London, British Institute of Learning Disabilities.

Weller, B. & Wells, R. (1990) *Baillière's Nurses' Dictionary*. London, Baillière Tindall Ltd.

Wiseman, T., Lowton, K. & Noonan, I. (2008) Transitions in the ageing population *in* Clarke, L. & Griffiths, P. (2008) *Learning Disability and Other Intellectual Impairments*. Chichester, John Wiley & Sons.

12

CARE AND SUPPORT FOR THOSE WHO ARE INFORMAL CARE GIVERS

The aims of this chapter are to highlight:

- The meaning of informal care giving

- The 'demographics' of informal care giving

- The experiences of those who are informal care givers

- Care giver legislation

- The roles of the nurse in supporting informal care givers.

By the end of this chapter you will be able to understand and discuss:

- The meaning of informal care giving

- The numbers, percentages, gender and ages of those giving informal care

- The personal experiences of those caring for a family member who has a learning disability

- The existence and impact of care giver legislation

- The role of the nurse in supporting those who are informal care givers.

PAUSE FOR THOUGHT 12.1

'I shouldn't have to spend my life proving that my son can't do things, to get the support my family needs to help him do things for himself.'

INTRODUCTION

Up to now, the focus of this book has been on those with a learning disability and their needs. In previous generations, those with a learning disability lived within specialist learning disability hospitals such as South Ockendon hospital in Essex, where I trained as a nurse in the last third of the 1980s. When these hospitals finally closed their doors in the 1990s, those with a learning disability were cared for within small community-based homes, a practice that was in line with official government policy of the day.

As a result of the closure of these long-stay hospitals, many people with a learning disability now live with and are cared for by their own families, a reality that may place an extra share of caring responsibility on these families. Therefore, the focus of this chapter will shift to these families, these 'informal care givers', and their experiences of caring for a person with a learning disability. Whilst much of this chapter will focus on issues that are pertinent to all care givers rather than care givers of those with a learning disability, parallels and implications will be made apparent for those caring for a family member who has a learning disability. I am indebted here to the *British Journal of Health Care Assistants* for their kind permission in allowing the use of definitions and statistics as they had been used in a series of articles written by me on care givers.

WHAT IS 'INFORMAL CARE GIVING'?

There are a number of issues around not so much the definition of informal care and carers but rather the language that is used. Some carers get rather angry at being called 'informal', saying that there is nothing informal about what they do. Often, the term 'care giver' is preferred to that of 'informal carer' and will be used throughout this chapter. So, what is this thing called 'care' and who are 'care givers' anyway? What is the difference between these and 'formal care' and 'formal carers'?

Formal carers are those who are employed, paid, trained and often regulated to provide care to another. This will include care professionals such as doctors, nurses, HCAs, social workers, professionals allied to medicine and religious ministers. Formal care is any care services that are provided by these care professionals in their professional lives.

In contrast, *care givers* (or *informal carers*) are those who provide care and support to a family member such as a parent, a sibling or a child with a disability or a friend in any care setting. This care is provided free, without pay, regulation and often without training, although there are an increasing number and variety of workshops, conferences and short training courses relevant and available for care givers. Examples of care givers include parents, partners, children, siblings, aunts, uncles, grandparents and friends.

A more formal definition of care givers may look like the following:

> "A carer is a person of any age, adult or child, who provides unpaid support to a partner, child, relative or friend who could not manage to live independently or whose health or wellbeing would deteriorate without this help. This could be due to frailty, disability or serious health condition, mental ill health or substance misuse"

> (RCGP, 2012)

In many ways, the roles of the care giver and the care professional overlap and it will not be unusual for care givers to carry out nursing roles such as wound or pain management. It is not unusual for care givers to be formal care professionals as well.

There are around 6.5 million care givers in the UK, which is 11% of the UK population, given a population of 60 million between the four countries of the UK (England, Scotland, Wales and Northern Ireland) (Carers UK, 2014). Care givers come from both genders with a gender split of around 58% female and 42% male (Princess Royal Trust for Carers, 2012). Care givers come from all ethnic backgrounds and cultures and from all ages from young children aged 7 or 8 who are caring for a sick or disabled sibling or parent to people who are in their 80s or 90s caring for a partner with dementia. Care givers come from all social backgrounds: from the then leader of the parliamentary opposition, David Cameron, who cared for his son before he died in 2009, to those living anonymously below the 'poverty line'. Those with a learning disability may also be care givers looking after a disabled or elderly parent.

- 1.5 million care givers care for more than 50 hours a week (RCGP, 2012)
- 68% of all care givers are of working age (RCGP, 2012)
- 1.2 million (20%) of all care givers give up paid employment in order to fulfil their caring responsibilities. Carer's allowance was less than £60 per week in 2014 and to qualify for carer's allowance, the care giver must be caring for at least 35 hours a week and can only earn an extra £100 per week through paid employment (HM Government, 2012a). This could, therefore, potentially have a significant impact upon family income and could even lead to family poverty. To put this into perspective, this means that the care giver 'earns' less than £2 per hour from the carer's allowance, bearing in mind that the national minimum wage in 2014 was £6.08 for those aged over 20 (HM Government, 2012b). There is anecdotal suggestion that those in paid employment often find that their promotion prospects are hindered although this would be illegal under the 2010 Equalities Act
- In 87% of households with working age carers looking after their partners, no one in that household is in paid employment (RCGP, 2012)
- For every hour per day every day that is spent in caring, the care giver saves the UK economy £6570 a year (Carers UK, 2011). Thus, if a care giver cares for 50 hours a week (7 hours per day every day) the annual amount of money that is saved to the UK economy becomes £46 000
- The amount that is saved to the UK economy by carers is £119 billion annually (Carers UK, 2011)
- 7% of care givers care for someone with a learning disability (Ouldred and Bryant, 2008)
- An estimated 25% of those with a learning disability are not known to social services (Ouldred and Bryant, 2008)
- Although the data are 20 years out of date, the incidence of depression in care givers is estimated at between 18 and 47% (Rosenthal *et al.*, 1993; Teri and Truax, 1994).

EXPERIENCES OF THOSE WHO ARE CARE GIVERS

During many informal conversations held with care givers over a number of years in a number of environments, views regarding how these care givers perceived the input and care by care professionals were aired. All of these views were anecdotal in nature and were written down as and when they occurred naturally, although those making these anecdotal comments were aware that I was a nurse. Most of these care professionals were nurses. Whilst a small number of these comments were positive and complementary of the care professionals whom care givers had engaged with, most, however, were angry and frustrated. Many of these conversations can be distilled down to the comments that are contained in the following tables. Whilst the vast majority of these comments appear negative, no attempt to edit these have been made as these represent the raw and often painful but real experiences of care givers. To so edit these comments would downplay and invalidate these experiences. (All these comments were made by people who are care givers who are supporting and caring for their family members or friends whilst accessing health care services).

> 'The support that I get from nurses, care staff, doctors, in fact all the ward staff is absolutely brilliant. They understand my son's needs, my needs as his father and have time for him and are able to communicate with him'.

Although the anecdotal comments that form the basis of this section were collected over a number of years from quite a large number of people, the above comment appears to be a rarity in its positive view of the support that a care giver received from care professionals, particularly nurses.

> 'When my son, who has autism, developed tonsillitis (which was a common occurrence) I phoned my GP for antibiotics. The agency GP practice nurse whom I spoke to said that it was flu, could not be bothered to look at my son's medical notes and put the phone down on me when I asked her to look at and read them.'
>
> 'My GP does not want to know.'
>
> 'Despite me being very stressed and my local GP practice nurse knowing that I am a full time care giver, this practice nurse either did not realise and understand how stressful and sometimes lonely being a care giver is or just could not be bothered. Either way, she passed up an excellent opportunity to ask how I was coping and, indeed, whether I was coping.'

These three comments highlight a perception, perhaps all too common, by some care givers that they are isolated and ignored by their GPs or GP practice nurses. However, increasing numbers of GP practices are compiling a register of care givers within their patch and promoting care giver assessments and support for those on this register. Therefore the support experienced by care givers who access GP services should improve.

> 'I receive no respite care'.
>
> 'I am on-call 24:7'.
>
> 'There is nothing left of me'.

Again, these three comments that speak of tiredness and exhaustion are all too common in the lives of care givers. Such exhaustion can and in many instances does lead to burn-out and declining physical, emotional and mental health in the care giver, and consequently to a decrease in ability to care.

> 'The nurses do not understand'.
>
> 'The nurses do not have the time to read my daughter's notes'.
>
> 'I have to do everything for my daughter when she has to go into hospital'.

Nursing and medical staff do not appear to have the training or ability to provide compassionate understanding, care and support to those with a learning disability and their care givers within NHS facilities such as a hospital ward. Consider whether appropriate, correct and safe care and treatment can be offered to any patient, whether learning disabled or not, if that patient's care/case notes are not read.

> 'I received only 15 minutes' training on how to give morphine injections to my adult son who has cancer'.
>
> 'I have attended a one day workshop on autism and I know everything that there is to know about this disorder' (*comment made by a social worker in the presence of a parent of a teenager with autism*).

These comments relate to issues around appropriate training for both care givers and care professionals. In relation to the first of these, consider how long it takes to train a student nurse to administer paracetamol to a patient without being supervised. Inappropriate training of care professionals and care givers could lead to very unsafe practices (15 minutes' training on how to administer morphine).

> 'When I accompanied my daughter who has a learning disability, and who was threatening to overdose on prescribed painkillers, to our local A&E department at no point did the A&E nursing staff take me to one side and allow me to talk, to unburden myself, to cry let alone give me any support'.
>
> 'There is very little out there to help me'.
>
> 'There is no place to rest and have a tea or coffee whilst in hospital supporting my daughter'.

These three comments speak of the care givers' need for emotional and psychological support for themselves, care and support which should be freely available, and their near-desperation when such support is not available or offered. These comments speak also of missed opportunities by nursing staff to reach out to, support and assist care givers.

> 'No one communicates'.
>
> 'The nursing and medical staff do not ask me or listen to me. I am not included in the care of my son despite the fact that I know my son and his needs better than they do'.
>
> 'I am ignored by the nursing staff whilst I am with my son in hospital'.

The key points here appear to be the feeling of being ignored, of not being listened to by care professionals or included as a valued member of the multi-disciplinary care team, and a lack of communication between care professionals and care givers.

It may be that these remarks made by care givers are little more than 'local gripes' that would not be replicated elsewhere and therefore are unfair and unjust. However, it may also be that these remarks may well be universal and therefore must stand as a sad comment on how care givers are viewed and treated by care professionals.

CARE GIVER LEGISLATION AND STRATEGY

There has been over the past two decades a growing realisation that the needs of care givers go largely unrecognised and unmet. In order to address this, a number of Acts of Parliament have been passed. All of these can be downloaded, free of charge, from the official Houses of Parliament website (see *References and Resources*) and www.legislation.gov.uk/.

Carers (Recognition and Services) Act 1995: The Carers Act 1995, as it is more commonly known, came into force on 1 April 1996 and was the first such legislation in the UK that specifically recognised the existence of care givers. Under this Parliamentary Act, individuals who provide or intend to provide a substantial amount of care on a regular basis are entitled to request an assessment of their ability to carry out and to continue to carry out that care. This assessment is carried out at the same time and was likely to form a part of the service user assessment.

Carers and Disabled Children Act 2000: The Carers and Disabled Children Act 2000 applies to care givers over 16 years of age and made the following principal changes to the existing 1995 Carers Act:

- It gave local councils mandatory duties to support care givers by providing services to care givers directly
- It gave care givers the right to an assessment independent of the person they care for
- It empowered local authorities to make direct payments to care givers
- It enabled councils to support flexibility in provision of short breaks through the short breaks voucher scheme.

Carers (Equal Opportunities) Act 2004: The first key area of this Act was that it imposed a duty on local and health authorities not only to provide care givers with an assessment (the 1995 Act) that was independent of any assessment, needs and wishes of the cared for (the 2000 Act), but also to inform care givers of their rights to such an assessment. The problem still remained, however, that local social services, councils and health authorities were largely unaware of exactly who or where the care givers were. That was due, in part, to care givers not making themselves known as such to local social services or GP practices. The second key issue within the Act was the recognition that many, if not most, care givers would like and even need paid employment and a social life outside of their care giving role.

Carers at the Heart of 21ˢᵗ Century Families and Communities 2008: This was expected to deliver genuine equality and recognition for care givers:

- Care givers to have a life of their own outside of caring
- Care givers to be supported so they did not suffer financial hardship as a result of their care giver responsibilities
- Care givers to be respected as expert care providers
- A 'social contract' called for the setting out of the responsibilities and expectations of the State, employers and care givers
- Care givers to be supported to remain physically and mentally healthy.

Recognised, Valued and Supported: Next Steps for the Carers Strategy 2010:

- The Coalition Government to work with care givers and care giver organisations to ease the burden of care giving
- Provision of £40 million over the following 4 years (which works out at £6.66 in total over the four years or £1.66 each year for each of the 6 million care givers in the UK) Four priority areas were identified, in collaboration with care givers and care giver organisations:
  - Supporting those with caring responsibilities to identify themselves as care givers
  - Enabling those with care giver responsibilities to fulfil their employment and educational potential
  - Personalised support for both cared for and care giver
  - Supporting care givers to remain mentally and physically well.

It could be argued from the above that legislative support for care givers began from an arguably grudging social service-led assessment of care givers' needs and abilities as an aspect of the assessment of the patient or service user, with the duty to request such an assessment resting solely with the care giver. However, the care giver was unlikely to ask for an assessment of their own needs if they did not know that they could. Care giver legislation as it now stands states that the care giver has the right to have an assessment of their needs independent of any assessment of the person they care for and independent of the wishes of the cared for. Local authorities have a legal duty to inform care givers of their rights and to inform them in such a way that meets the information requirements of the care giver. However, this is not the same as those care giver needs, once assessed, being appropriately met!

THE ROLES OF THE NURSE

CASE STUDY 12.1

Jill, whom we met towards the end of *Chapter 9*, works at a GP practice as a health care assistant and at a local community health centre. Whilst working within these settings with a number of patients and service users who have a learning disability, she comes into regular contact with a number of their families. Consequently, Jill has developed an interest in supporting these families to meet their own needs.

There are a number of supportive roles that Jill can engage in that would meet the needs of those who are care givers. The Foundation for People with Learning Disabilities (2002) suggested that care givers should be offered practical and emotional support, respite breaks, access to support groups and independent advocacy. Care givers should be offered advice regarding planning for the future. Whilst these make for good starting points, where exactly does Jill start?

A good starting point for Jill would be to gain a working knowledge of the prevalence, gender mix, age range of and main issues affecting care givers in general, along with a working knowledge of care giver legislation and national, regional and local care giver strategies. This would require awareness of and access to care giver organisations such as Carers UK (www.carersuk.org) and the Princess Royal Trust for Carers (www.carers.org) for information and advice. Jill could become a member of either of these two organisations as a way of keeping herself informed and up to date with current issues affecting care givers. Local care giver organisations are usually very willing to do short presentations to care professionals. Jill should not forget that those with a learning disability may also be care givers themselves, as well as being care recipients, in so far as they could be the primary care giver for an elderly or disabled parent. As such they are likely to need extra support both as a person with a learning disability *and* as a care giver.

On a practical level, Jill could:

- Ensure that all GP and health centre appointments and appointment times, whether for the care giver or the person cared for, take into account the needs of the care giver and cared for rather than the needs of the service.
- Ask the right questions of the care giver and listen carefully without judging either the care giver or the answers. Remember that the care giver is likely to know more about caring for someone with a learning disability than Jill does!
- Make time during any consultation with the care giver so that the care giver does not feel rushed and that he or she feels valued, validated, listened to and understood.
- Provide clear, accurate and up-to-date information regarding a wide range of issues that are pertinent to care givers and in a format that is accessible for care givers. This format could be either written or verbal, in English or a wide variety of community languages, from academic journal articles to 'easy read'.
- Be involved in care giver assessments as part of a multi-disciplinary team.
- Advocate on behalf of family care givers in the provision of equipment, carers' grants, welfare benefits and respite care, amongst many others. Respite care may not necessarily be planned weekend breaks from the responsibilities of care giving but may also include someone going into the family's home (home respite) for a couple of hours so that the care giver can have some 'me time', spend time with other people or go shopping.
- Help to set up and facilitate care giver support groups at the health centre where she works. This may simply involve booking the meeting room and speakers, providing basic admin support and refreshments, and being available to answer care givers' questions.

Those nurses who work in surgical or medical wards or, for that matter, any ward within a general acute hospital could offer care givers who spend significant time at the hospital caring for and supporting their family member or friend the opportunity to use the staff room for 'comfort breaks'. After all, you would not like the idea of working an entire shift without taking a coffee break; neither do care givers!

CONCLUSION

Care givers can often be faced with a daunting task that could involve working or being available '24/7' and often without appropriate support from health and social care professionals. Yet, it can often be these same care professionals to whom care givers turn for help and support and it can often be these care professionals who identify that care givers are in need of support and what that support is likely to be. If in doubt, remember that the NMC's code of professional conduct places a professional duty on all nurses to communicate and work collaboratively with all members of the multi-disciplinary team **including patients / service users and their families**.

KEY POINTS

- There are 6 million care givers in the UK, i.e. 10% of the current UK population.

- A care giver is a person of any age, adult or child, who provides unpaid support to a partner, child, relative or friend who could not manage to live independently or whose health or wellbeing would deteriorate without this help.

- Many care givers are likely to have negative experiences of support and care at the hands of care professionals.

- There are a number of Parliamentary Acts that serve to meet the diverse needs of care givers.

- The role of the nurse includes listening to and providing accurate information to care givers, the provision of care giver friendly services as well as assisting in the setting up and facilitation of care giver support groups.

REFERENCES AND RESOURCES

Carers UK (2014) *Why we're here*. Available at: http://www.carersuk.org/about-us/why-we-re-here (last accessed 16 November 2014)

Foundation for People with Learning Disabilities (2002) *Charter of rights for older people with learning disabilities and family carers*. London, FPLD.

HM Government (2012a) *Carer's allowance*. Available at: www.direct.gov.uk/en/moneytaxandbenefits/benefitstaxcreditsandothersupport/caringforsomeone/dg_10018705 (last accessed 16 October 2014)

HM Government (2012b) *National Minimum Wage rates*. Available at: www.direct.gov.uk/en/employment/employees/thenationalminimumwage/dg_10027201 (last accessed 16 October 2014)

Houses of Parliament website: www.parliament.uk/business/bills-and-legislation/acts-of-parliament/ (last accessed 11 November 2014)

Ouldred, E. & Bryant, C. (2008) The older adult, intellectual impairments and the dementias. *In* Clark, L. & Griffiths, P. (2008) *Learning Disability and Other Intellectual Impairments*. Chichester, John Wiley & Sons.

Princess Royal Trust for Carers (2012) *Key Facts about Carers*. Available at www.carers.org/key-facts-about-carers (last accessed 16 October 2014)

Rosenthal, C., Sulman, J. & Marshall, V. (1993) Depressive symptoms in family care givers of long stay patients. *Gerontologist*, 33: 249–56.

Royal College of General Practitioners / Princess Royal Trust for Carers (2012) *Supporting Carers: an action guide for general practitioners and their teams (second edition)*. London, RCGP.

Teri, L. & Truax, P. (1994) Assessment of depression in dementia patients: association of caregiver mood with depression ratings. *Gerontologist*, 34: 231–234.

13

DISABILITY AND CARER DISCRIMINATION

AIMS AND LEARNING OUTCOMES:

The aims of this chapter are to highlight:

- Those who are experience learning disabilities either as service users, care givers or care professionals and their experiences of disability discrimination

- The roles of the nurse in tackling disability discrimination.

By the end of this chapter you will be able to understand:

- The impact that disability discrimination can have on those with a learning disability and their families

- Your roles as a nurse and a citizen in tackling disability discrimination.

PAUSE FOR THOUGHT 13.1

Disability discrimination is a hate crime: discuss.

INTRODUCTION

It could be suggested that those with a learning disability have endured a very long history of discrimination on the grounds of their disability and societal responses to this disability. Such discrimination arguably begins prior to birth and, again arguably, lasts until after the person has died. Family members as care givers are also likely to experience discrimination due to their association with the person with a learning disability (disability by proxy) (see *Chapter 12* for a more detailed exposition of potential care giver discrimination). In this, those with a learning disability are not alone as they are likely to share a common history of discrimination with those who have physical disability issues or mental health issues or are lesbian, gay, bisexual or transgender. These are the claims and issues that are central to this chapter.

We have previously met Jill (an HCA who works in her local GP practice and community health centre and who has a sibling with Down's syndrome), Marcel (a '30-something' man with Down's syndrome), Ziva (Marcel's sister, who also has Asperger's syndrome) and Hanif (a second-year student nurse who works in a hospital medical ward). They would now like to invite you to engage in a conversation with them regarding their experiences of disability discrimination. **The views and beliefs expressed here by these four participants are highly subjective and personal and must be viewed accordingly.**

WHAT IS DISCRIMINATION?

Marcel: Welcome one and all to my humble abode and thanks for taking the time out of your all too busy days to be here. Help yourselves to the tea, coffee, biscuits and cakes. The cakes and biscuits are provided by my darling sister Ziva who I believe baked them herself!

Ziva: Thanks for the invite, Marcel. Now, disability discrimination is not an easy thing to understand let alone talk about. I think that it may be helpful here to understand what discrimination actually is before we go on to discuss how this thing called discrimination affects us. Is that OK? So, Hanif, what do you understand by the term disability discrimination?

Hanif: As I neither have a disability myself nor have a family member who does have a disability, I have the dubious luxury of being able to look in from outside, so to speak, to be able to see both the 'trees' and the 'wood' in terms of disability issues, including disability discrimination. I would like to say that I don't have a clue as to the meaning of disability discrimination but that would be cheating! To me, disability discrimination means to treat one person differently from another on the grounds of the person's disability.

Jill: That's as fine as it goes, Hanif, but I think that there is much more to the term 'discrimination' than that! After all, I engage, interact and communicate with, and therefore treat my boss differently from the way I do my husband or my friends down at the pub. This is only right and proper as this involves both professional and personal boundaries. Is this discrimination though? I don't think that it is. So, can you explain further what disability discrimination means for you?

Hanif: Sorry about that Jill and, yes, I do get your point although I did add "*on the grounds of that person's disability*". Is discrimination where one person is treated not so much differently but either better or worse than another person on the basis of certain characteristics?

Jill: You've got it about right! There is positive discrimination, where one person is offered more favourable opportunities and conditions than another in order to allow the first person to engage and compete within certain aspects of society and socio-economic life such as employment and education. Positive discrimination allows for a 'level playing field' that permits all people to engage in socially valued activities. However, negative discrimination is: "The act of denying rights, benefits, justice, equitable treatment, or access to facilities available to all others, to an individual or group of people because of their race, age, gender, handicap or other defining characteristic" (Megson, 2011).

Hanif: That seems to be fairly straightforward, although I take issue with Megson's use of the word 'handicap'. I thought that this particular word and its historical socio-political baggage had been confined to the history books.

Marcel: I agree with that. To me, many people because they are old, fat, poor, unemployed, disabled, black, Asian, or a single or teenage mum can be discriminated against. Often, some people don't need a reason to be unkind and hate another person; it is just the way that they are and it is so sad!

Ziva: In terms of discrimination and employment, discrimination against a disabled employee occurs if, on the grounds of that employee's disability, the employee is treated less favourably than an employee not having that particular disability whose relevant circumstances are the same or not materially different from those of the disabled person. This, by the way, is taken from the 2010 Equality Act.

Jill: I know that this may be cheating, but realising what we were going to discuss this evening I took the liberty of looking up the word 'discrimination' on the internet and found this little nugget on Wikipedia. Although using Wikipedia as a source of information may be frowned upon because some entries may be less than accurate, I think that it is worth quoting in full: "**Discrimination** is the prejudicial and/or distinguishing treatment of an individual based on their actual or perceived membership in a certain group or category, 'in a way that is worse than the way people are usually treated'. It involves the group's initial reaction or interaction, influencing the individual's actual behavior towards the group or the group leader, restricting members of one group from opportunities or privileges that are available to another group, leading to the exclusion of the individual or entities based on logical or irrational decision making. Discriminatory traditions, policies, ideas, practices, and laws exist in many countries and institutions in every part of the world, even in ones where discrimination is generally looked down upon. In some places, controversial attempts such as quotas or affirmative action have been used to benefit those believed to be current or past victims of discrimination—but have sometimes been called reverse discrimination themselves" (http://en.wikipedia.org/wiki/Discrimination)

Marcel: There is an awful lot there! Is there any chance that we can unpack some of this so that I could understand it better?

Jill: Well, the first part of this definition is fairly simple and it just repeats what we have already said about discrimination. By 'being a member of a certain group or category' is meant being young, old, black, Asian, disabled, etc. The last part of this definition suggests that although largely discredited, discriminatory practices still exist under various guises such as 'affirmative action'.

Hanif: OK, but the middle section confuses me. I get it that discrimination is based on one person's or group's view and thus response to, and interaction with another person or group on the grounds of difference, whether perceived or real, and that such responses and interactions are often irrational. Is that what Wikipedia is getting at here?

Jill: Yes, I think so.

EXPERIENCES OF THOSE WHO HAVE A LEARNING DISABILITY

"A few years ago, I was near my house with my fiancée on our way to the day centre when some school children started chucking stones at us. They had followed me before. They were calling us names. They called my fiancée a name as well, saying racist things 'cos she's white and the boys were black. We were shocked, upset and angry. I went to the police, but they were not very helpful. They didn't arrest anyone.

I still see them sometimes in the street. They go their way and I go my way, but I am still worried by what could happen. I still think the police should have done more at the time to make sure this can't happen again.

Hate crime upsets me. When I hear people affected by it, it brings back painful memories. I have still got emotional scars (a scar in the mind) from my experience".

('Neil's story': Mencap, 2013a)

Hanif: You make a number of interesting observations, Marcel. You are right that discrimination is not limited to people with disabilities. People who are lesbian, gay, bisexual or transgender, from a different cultural or ethnic background or those who experience mental health problems have had to endure decades of discrimination. Similarly, one has only to observe the taunting, teasing and downright bullying that school children engage in and are victims of. Anyone who looks or sounds different in any way appears to be fair game. You only have to be too tall, too short, too thin, too fat, wear glasses or have freckles or spots to be subject to discrimination and bullying.

Ziva: I agree. You only have to look at 'Neil's story' that is presented by Mencap to realise how looking, sounding, behaving and just being different can give rise to bullying and discrimination by other people. Marcel, have you experienced bullying and discrimination similar to Neil?

Marcel: No I haven't, Ziva, but I do know people who have! Friends of mine have been called names and have been sworn at by school children and it is so sad to see even young children have such fear and hatred of those who are different.

Ziva: To change the subject a bit, with the increase of internet bullying and discrimination has also come an increase in victims of such bullying and discrimination engaging in acts of self-harm and even suicide. So it is not just those with disabilities that are likely to be subject to negative discrimination with often disastrous results.

Jill: I came across a number of newspaper articles recently that appear to confirm the often painful nature of actual or perceived discrimination. The first concerns a mother who kills her 12-year-old autistic son by throwing him off the Humber Bridge and then commits suicide by following him (Wainwright, 2006). The second concerns a young lady with a learning disability who was bullied and made to carry out absolutely horrendous acts by those who she thought were her friends. These so-called friends eventually murdered her (Mencap, 2011).

Marcel: Thanks for raising these issues, Jill. I have not heard of the first of these although it does not surprise me at all! I often feel isolated, very lonely and vulnerable as a result of my learning disability. Although it may seem to you that I am fairly self-confident and able, I still experience poor or non-existent services and support by care staff who don't seem to care and can't be bothered, who don't want to know. Is that discrimination? I think that it is. Whether that would lead to me killing myself, probably not but I can understand why in extreme cases some people would. Disability discrimination as a hate crime: now that's a different matter. Yes, I am very familiar with this and so are many of my friends. I have many friends who have been bullied, sworn at, punched, kicked, called names and spat at for no other reason than that they have a learning disability.

Ziva: I know what you mean, Marcel. I checked the Mencap website (www.mencap.org.uk/search/apachesolr_search/hate%20crime) before I came here this evening and there are dozens of articles on disability discrimination as hate crimes. Most of those who are victims of hate crimes share that they are still mentally and emotionally scarred. Many of these are still too afraid to even leave their homes for fear of what might happen to them. I believe that disability discrimination can cause symptoms that are pretty close to post-traumatic stress disorder.

Hanif: Hang on a minute! I thought that disability discrimination is illegal under the 2010 Equality Act, at least in public / professional life!

Marcel: Is it really? You could have fooled me! Disability discrimination may well be against the law but it still happens. I will give you an example: a local politician in Cornwall, Collin Brewer (Mencap, 2013b) stated that children with a disability are like deformed lambs and should be killed by throwing them against a brick wall. He believed that the money that would be saved through the killing of disabled children would open and run ten public toilets. I am worth less than a public toilet! This makes me sick, angry and very scared. Words cannot begin to describe how I feel about this! I cried for hours when I heard this! Is this Mr. Brewer the only one to think like this? I don't think that he is and I am petrified!

Ziva: I know how you feel, Marcel. Don't forget that I have Asperger's syndrome and that Brewer's comments are also directed at me and those like me. I am extremely worried as I don't believe that Brewer is alone in believing that you and I are trash. To me, such views impact on all of us in many ways.

Jill: What do you mean by that? Again, surely Brewer was 'last year's news'. Have we not moved on since then?

Ziva: I will answer your second question first, Jill. Yes, Brewer was last year. Have we moved on since then? No! An interesting news snippet caught my eye only a few days ago: Conservative councillor and mayor of Swindon, Nick Martin, 63, was found guilty of breaching the members' code of conduct after Labour complained about comments he made last year. Labour councillors said they heard him say: "*Are we still letting Mongols* [people with Down's syndrome] *have sex with each other?*" (www.bbc.co.uk/news/uk-england-wiltshire-27034445 and www.theguardian.com/commentisfree/2014/apr/15/hard-life-disabled-hating-bigot-mayor). I believe that such ignorance is rather widespread. To answer your first question, I believe that on the level of society, disability discrimination makes us all poorer. It brutalises and dehumanises us, as can be seen by Brewer's and Martin's comments. I believe that discrimination engenders and perpetuates discrimination and with that, the willingness to destroy those who are in any way different. It is almost a crime to be different in today's world.

Hanif: Strong words, Ziva. Do you have anything to back up your arguments?

Ziva: One word: eugenics. Although the ideas and practice of eugenics that was so prevalent in the first half of the 20th century has largely been discredited, there is a rather interesting snippet in a recent edition of the *Nursing Standard* (Pearce, 2013) where a foetus was aborted for no other reason than having a cleft lip.

Hanif: That is a rather tenuous link, Ziva. It is also very emotive and, although I can understand how and why you feel like this, we are perhaps straying from the main issue under discussion here, that of the effects that disability discrimination has on people.

Ziva: Point taken. However, to continue my train of thought for a moment, I believe that disability discrimination affects care professionals and those discriminated against, as well as society. Disability discrimination demeans, brutalises, impoverishes and dehumanises care professionals and can often lead to stress and burnout and the possibility of abuse. Disability discrimination, indeed any form of discrimination, could lead to the nurse being in breach of the Nursing and Midwifery Council's code of professional conduct (NMC, 2008) and this would therefore be grounds for professional misconduct charges. In relation to those with disabilities, as has already been mentioned, I believe that discrimination leads to rejection, humiliation, fear, intimidation, isolation, loneliness, anger and even in extreme cases the destruction and extinction of the person. I know that these are harsh and emotive words, particularly when I suggest that an effect of disability discrimination can lead to the destruction and extinction of the person. However, picking up on the *Nursing Standard* article that I have just mentioned, that is what I meant by suggesting that a foetus was aborted on the grounds of having a cleft lip, a cleft lip that could easily be rectified through minor surgery.

Marcel: I think I understand what you are saying, Ziva. I have watched with great pain and sadness the TV programmes on Winterbourne View. Those with a learning disability were treated as trash by those whose job it was to care for them. I don't believe that Winterbourne View was the only care home or hospital where my friends were discriminated against to the point of abuse and torture on the grounds of their learning disability. What kind of world are we living in that turns its back on such abuse and discrimination and allows it to happen?

THE ROLES OF THE NURSE

Jill: That is a very sad thing to say, Marcel…

Marcel: Yes Jill, I know it is, but to me it's true and real! The question is: what are you and Hanif as nurses going to do about it? Is there anything that you and other nurses can do?

Jill: I think that there are a number of things that I and my colleagues can do as health care professionals. For a start we need to be aware of our own personal biases, prejudices, beliefs, social attitudes and world views. We are only human, we are not machines and we will, whether we like it or not, have our own prejudices, beliefs and attitudes. The trick is to acknowledge them and how they can impact upon the care and support services that we offer. Following on from that we need to be aware of and reflect upon the biases, beliefs, prejudices and attitudes in others and how these impact upon the lives of those around us.

Hanif: I agree; we need to be aware of the personal and societal attitudes and beliefs of those who worked at places like Winterbourne View and that led to the horrendous treatment of those living at these places. If we are not aware of and do not understand these attitudes and beliefs we are condemned to not only holding these same views and prejudices, but acting upon them.

Ziva: I would need you as care professionals to be aware of, understand and implement organisational policies on anti-discrimination. I am well aware that there will be a rather large folder full of policies, procedures and guidelines that will cover many aspects of how the nurse works on a daily basis such as health and safety, manual handling, safe handling and administration of medicines, what to do in a fire and so on. At the very least you should be aware of where these policies and procedures are kept and have read many of them during your induction period. Policies on anti-discriminatory behaviour should form a crucial aspect of this policy folder.

Jill: I would also expect nurses and other health care professionals to be fully aware of and understand both the contents and the underlying philosophy of the 2010 Equalities Act and how this Act seeks to tackle discrimination in all its forms. I notice that we have not discussed any of the human rights legislation that is relevant to those with disabilities such as the Human Rights Act, the Disability Discrimination Act 1995 and the Equalities Act 2010. Is there any reason for this omission?

Ziva: Yes Jill, you are right. However, the short answer is lack of space and time for a meaningful discussion on anti-discrimination legislation here. The laws that you just mentioned are vital to a proper understanding of, and debate around disability discrimination. Such a debate could well form the basis of a further chapter to this book but is too complex to be covered here. Sorry about that!

Hanif: That's OK! I have always found that active participation in professional development opportunities such as short courses and workshops, discussions with colleagues and research to be a very good way of raising my own knowledge around discriminatory issues.

Marcel: If you do discriminate, be willing and prepared to justify your attitudes and behaviours and accept their consequences. You must also be prepared and willing to challenge discriminatory practice both within yourself and within others.

Jill: Good point, Marcel. Nurses are governed by the Nursing and Midwifery Council's code of professional conduct. Read, understand and abide by this code. Finally, I would recommend that whatever you do, record and report any forms of discrimination that you encounter.

CONCLUSION

Discrimination of those with various disabilities on the grounds of their disability has been a 'fixture' in many people's lives for decades, if not centuries. Whilst disability discrimination in many areas of life is now illegal under the 2010 Equalities Act, those with a learning disability still experience discrimination, as Marcel and his friends demonstrate. As a nurse, you have a primary duty to do no harm. This duty must include recognising and challenging disability discrimination wherever and whenever it is found. Not to do so results in colluding in such discrimination. Always remember, disability discrimination, whatever form it takes, is a hate crime and must be challenged as such.

KEY POINTS

- Discrimination involves the act of denying rights, benefits, justice, equitable treatment, or access to facilities available to all others, to an individual or group of people because of their race, age, gender, handicap or other defining characteristic.

- Disability discrimination, although illegal, still continues in many environments and by many people including care staff (e.g. Winterbourne View) and politicians.

- Disability discrimination can be seen as a hate crime which can cause severe psychological and emotional harm to the victim.

- The role of the nurse includes being aware of and understanding personal beliefs and attitudes to those with a learning disability, being aware of and understanding employer policies and anti-discrimination legislation and challenging discrimination when and where it occurs.

REFERENCES

Megson, D. (2011) Discrimination against disabilities: a life worth less? *British Journal of Healthcare Assistants*, 5:10; 495–498.

Mencap (2011) *'Missed opportunities' in hate crime case*. Available at www.mencap.org.uk/news/article/missed-opportunities-hate-crime-case (last accessed 16 October 2014)

Mencap (2013a) *My experience of hate crime*. Available at: www.mencap.org.uk/blogs/my-experience-hate-crime (last accessed 16 October 2014)

Mencap (2013b) *Mencap calls for the resignation of Collin Brewer*. Available at: www.mencap.org.uk/news/article/mencap-calls-resignation-collin-brewer-0 (last accessed 16 October 2014)

Nursing and Midwifery Council (2008) *The Code: standards of conduct, performance and ethics for nurses and midwives*. Available at: www.nmc-uk.org/Documents/Standards/The-code-A4-20100406.pdf (last accessed 16 October 2014)

Pearce, L. (2013) Cleft palate services had to be reformed. *Nursing Standard*, 28:12; 23.

Wainwright, M. (2006) A mother and son smiling at the station. Then two specks on the edge of a bridge. *The Guardian*, 19 April. Available at: www.theguardian.com/uk/2006/apr/19/martinwainwright.mainsection

14

LEARNING DISABILITY AND SPIRITUALITY

AIMS AND LEARNING OUTCOMES:

The aims of this chapter are to highlight:

- The meaning of spirituality and the differences and similarities between spirituality and religion

- The barriers that prevent those with a learning disability from experiencing and expressing their spirituality

- The resources that are available that may assist those with a learning disability in experiencing and expressing their spiritual dimension

- How nurses can support those with a learning disability to experience and express their spirituality.

By the end of this chapter, you will be able to demonstrate an understanding of:

- The meaning of spirituality

- How spirituality is both similar to and different from religion

- The various barriers that could hinder or prevent those with a learning disability in engaging in and expressing their own spiritual identity

- The various resources that are available that could assist in a meaningful spiritual engagement, expression and identity

- How you as a nurse can assist those with a learning disability to so engage and express their spiritual identity.

INTRODUCTION

Much of this book has focused on perhaps the more physical aspects of working with and providing care and support for those with a learning disability. However, nurses must work within a holistic framework; they must plan, provide and assess and evaluate holistically. Spirituality is a vital component of such holistic care.

Spirituality is often appended to end of life care as very much an 'afterthought'. Even then it may not be with a great deal of understanding of the needs of the person or comprehension that spirituality is for the whole of life and not just at the end of that life. Swinton (2002) argued that the spirituality of people with learning disabilities is under-researched and frequently misunderstood. Barber (2013) argued that those with a learning disability have as great a spiritual need and as much right to have that need met as anyone else in society. This is the central argument in this chapter.

I am indebted here to the *British Journal of Health Care Assistants* for their very kind permission in allowing the use of definitions, meanings and barriers as they had been used in a series of articles written by me on spirituality.

WHAT IS SPIRITUALITY?

PAUSE FOR THOUGHT 14.1

Are you aware of, and comfortable with your own sense of the spiritual, with your own spiritual identity? Do you know what spirituality is and the similarities and differences between spirituality and religion?

What, then, is this thing called spirituality? Is it a thing or is it much more intimate and profound than that? How does spirituality manifest itself? Given that there may be some confusion between religion and spirituality, with these two concepts or phenomena appearing to mean the same thing, is spirituality the same as religion? What are its similarities with and differences to religion? In today's world, is spirituality relevant? Do I have the time, the ability and the resources to engage in another person's spirituality?

These and a hundred other questions spring to mind at the mere mention of spirituality. So what, then, is spirituality?

There are a wide range of meanings that can be given to the phenomenon of spirituality.

MacKinlay (2006, p. 13) suggests that:

"Spirituality is the personal quest for understanding answers to ultimate questions about life, about meaning and about relationships to the sacred or the transcendent which may (or may not) lead to or arise from the development of religious rituals".

MacKinlay (2006, p. 13) also suggests that spirituality refers to an ultimate meaning of self and life that is mediated through relationships with others and with God (however one defines this term), the environment, the arts and through religion.

In a survey of definitions conducted by McSherry (2007), the following was highlighted:

- "Spirituality is my inner being. It is who I am. It is me expressed through my body, my thinking and my feelings" (Stoll, 1989, p. 61)
- A quality that goes beyond religious affiliation, that strives for inspiration, reverence, awe, meaning and purpose. Spirituality can also be seen as a belief in a supernatural or divine force that has power over the universe and commands worship and obedience (Murray and Zentner, 1989, pp. 257 and 259)
- The way in which men and women may understand their existence and the action which comes from this understanding (Males and Boswell, 1990, p. 35)
- Spirituality refers to the propensity to make meaning through a sense relatedness to dimensions that transcend the self in such a way that empowers and does not devalue the individual (Reed, 1992, p. 350)
- Spirituality is a personal search for meaning and purpose in life which may or may not be related to religion. It entails connection to self-chosen and/or religious beliefs, values and practices that gives meaning to life (Tanyi, 2002, p. 506).

Again, Wiseman (2006, p. 4) follows Schneiders (1989) in suggesting that spirituality has three interrelated dimensions or references:

- Spirituality is a fundamental aspect of the human being and what it means to be human
- Spirituality is the lived experience that actualises this fundamental aspect of humanness
- Spirituality is the study of this lived experience.

However, it could be suggested that spirituality is different from religion, although many people confuse the two and consider religion and spirituality as the same thing. So what is religion?

MacKinlay (2006, p. 13) suggests that religion is "an organised system of beliefs, practices, rituals and symbols that is designed to facilitate closeness to the sacred or transcendent through fostering an understanding of one's relationship and responsibility to others in living together in a community". MacKinlay (2006, p. 13) goes on to say that religion is part of spirituality. The practice of religion is a way that humans relate to the sacred and to others.

Murray and Zentner (1989, p. 259) suggest that religion is "a system of beliefs, a comprehensive code of ethics or philosophy, a set of practices that are followed, a church affiliation, the conscious pursuit of any object the person holds as supreme".

Thus, spirituality could be seen as one way that an individual understands and connects to oneself, others, the world and the 'divine' (however one defines the divine), whilst religion provides a community and a structure that nurtures and provides a framework for this understanding and connectivity to take root and grow.

BARRIERS TO EXPERIENCING AND PRACTISING SPIRITUALITY

Those with a learning disability have the same right as anyone else to experience and express their own spiritual identity and to do so in ways that they feel comfortable with. However, it could be suggested that those with a learning disability face and experience barriers to such spiritual experiences and expression in much the same way that they do in other areas of life, as a result of having a learning disability.

What, then, are these barriers? Those with a learning disability could experience some, perhaps many, of the following:

- Spiritual and faith community support being a 'curate's egg', i.e. good in parts. Where it is good, it is very good and where it is bad it is bad!
- Those with learning disabilities are often ignored, patronised and treated as little children, regardless of whether the person is an adult with adult needs and life experiences
- Those with a learning disability are often lumped together as a homogenous group instead of being engaged with as an individual, and without taking into account the background, culture, abilities and wishes of individual service users (one size fits all!)
- Faith leaders and faith communities tend not to understand either learning disability as a concept or those with a learning disability
- Little genuine and sensitive help is offered, either by faith communities or health and social care staff, to support those with a learning disability to be comfortable with and express their own spirituality.

Here are a number of anecdotal experiences of some of those with a learning disability, gathered through a number of conversations:

- 'My priest does not understand me'
- 'The care staff where I live are too busy to make time to really be with me, to listen to me'
- 'The care staff where I live are embarrassed when I try to pray'
- 'The care staff where I live seem to find my attempts at prayer funny'
- 'I feel trapped in a system that does not care'
- 'Too much noise, too much busyness'
- 'I have no contact with my local mosque' (the same could apply equally to other faith communities)
- 'I am a Jew, but the only religious service that I can go to is run by the hospital-based Church of England vicar'
- 'I often feel ignored by my church'
- 'I feel that I am being treated as a little child'
- 'I feel lonely. Everyone talks to each other, but no-one talks to me'
- 'No-one helps me to talk to God'.

It could be that some of these barriers result from a lack of understanding of those with a learning disability by faith communities and their leaders, while others result from issues within the care environment.

Again, those with a learning disability may have been viewed as:

- Unable to engage in spirituality in any meaningful way, due to assumptions about their lack of ability to understand and reason (Gaventa, 2010)
- 'Holy and saintly simple people', as God's 'specially chosen'. As a result of this, those with a learning disability were often put on pedestals, adulated and out of the reach of 'ordinary' people. As a further result, those with a learning disability became outsiders
- The result of sin, either their own or, more likely, their parents' or grandparents' (see St. John's Gospel 9:2 for an example of this from the Christian tradition). This, again, has a similar 'outsider' effect. It was a popular idea and doctrine at the time the Christian Gospels were written and compiled, and in the Jewish faith and early Christian church, that all suffering, illness and disability in this life had their origins in sin, hence the suggestion in Jn 9:2 that the man was born blind as a result of his own or his parents' sin. This position has been discredited by biblical scholars for at least 50 years although there may be certain parts of the Christian tradition who would continue to uphold this interpretation (see the Andrew Womack Ministries website for a possible illustration of this; http://www.awmi.net/bible/joh_09_02.

All of these were likely to have a negative impact upon a spiritual identity that those with a learning disability could meaningfully own, experience and express.

SPIRITUAL RESOURCES

Having briefly highlighted a number of potential barriers that could impact upon and potentially prevent a person with a learning disability from meaningfully owning, experiencing and expressing their own authentic spirituality, are there any resources that could be of use to both those with a learning disability and to nurses? In answer to this question, the following range of resources (a range that is by no means exhaustive) may be useful. Some of these resources may be more helpful to those with a learning disability rather than nurses; the first three may fall into that category. The next two resources may be helpful to both those who have a learning disability and to nurses, whilst the remainder may be of more help to nurses than those with a learning disability.

Hospital chaplains

The hospital chaplaincy team are employed to provide spiritual and faith support to patients, service users, staff and patients' families. However, chaplains who have been appropriately trained in providing spiritual and faith community support to those with a learning disability may be of more immediate use and value to such patients during their stay in hospital than nurses. Key roles of the team and individual chaplains is to provide a link for the patient and staff between the hospital ward or clinical setting and the wide variety of faith communities, and to be a listening friend to patients and staff alike. They are also involved in the ongoing professional development of hospital staff regarding dignity, spirituality and faith communities. These teams can be contacted via the hospital switchboard and/or hospital chapel. The website for the College of Health Care Chaplains is www.healthcarechaplains.org.

Local faith communities

Those with a learning disability have as much right to attend and participate in the spiritual, liturgical, pastoral and social life of their preferred faith community as anyone else. Whilst most general acute hospitals will have a multi-faith chaplaincy team who will support patients and service users who have a learning disability, it would still be useful to forge links with the person's own faith community. This is so that such faith communities could maintain contact with the person whilst he or she is in hospital and ensure that the person with a learning disability is still included in the spiritual, liturgical and pastoral life of their faith community. This is particularly important if the person with a learning disability is likely to be in hospital for any length of time.

Jean Vanier and L'Arche

Vanier is a French–Canadian philosopher, theologian, prolific writer and humanitarian who, in 1964, invited two people who had learning disabilities to live with him in a small village in France. Out of this small and simple beginning grew L'Arche, an international network of small community homes for those with learning disabilities run on largely Christian lines. There are seven L'Arche communities in England (London, Ipswich, Preston, Manchester, Dover, Bognor and Liverpool), two in Scotland (Edinburgh and Inverness) and two in Wales (Cornerstone and the Brecon) (L'Arche, 2013). Alongside these communities exist 'faith and light' ecumenical faith groups (Faith and Light Communities, 2012) where those with learning disabilities and their friends and families come together to explore and engage in the spiritual dimension of the human journey (www.faithandlight.org.uk). Vanier's website is www.jean-vanier.org/en/home.

Mindfulness

The Buddhist-based practice of mindfulness exercises or mindfulness-based cognitive therapy (MBCT) are ways of paying attention to the present moment, using spiritual methods such as meditation, breathing and yoga (www.mentalhealth.org.uk/help-information/mental-health-a-z/M/mindfulness/). Mindfulness training, as a way of reducing stress, helps us become more aware of our thoughts and feelings so that instead of being overwhelmed by them, we are better able to manage them. In perhaps more practical terms, mindfulness is a way of being slowly and quietly but totally present and connected to the present moment and to the totality (mind, body and spirit) of both the self and other people within this moment in time.

John Swinton and Kairos

Kairos was established by John Swinton (professor of practical theology at the University of Aberdeen) and Christina Gangemi, to provide advice, information, advocacy, and support for individuals who have a learning disability and their families regarding spirituality, religious practice and the vital role that those with a learning disability and their families have within communities. The creation of a space for the development of networks of lay people, professionals and religious communities was seen as crucial as a way of providing information regarding spirituality and learning disability (The Kairos Forum, 2013).

Hospital guidelines and policies

Treating patients and service users with respect and dignity will form the cornerstone of most, if not all hospital, NHS Trust or other health and social care providers' policies and procedures. This will include policies on respecting the religious, faith and spiritual beliefs of all patients, service users and staff. It is likely that, during a new employee's induction period, they will either be given a complete set of these policies or be encouraged to locate and read these policies and will be expected to sign to say that they have read them. It is always good practice for established and experienced staff to similarly locate and read these policies, many of which will be updated over time.

Books and journal articles

There is a vast library of books, academic papers and conference presentations that explores the rich and varied meanings and lived experiences of spirituality, both as part of and outside of faith communities; too many to highlight here. There is also an increasing number of books and nursing journal articles/papers as well as conference presentations that focus on spirituality, religious faith and health care, as can be seen in the references given below. Many of these explore spirituality and faith community engagement of those who have a learning disability. These books and articles are well worth exploring further.

Slow nursing

Many nurses work in a highly pressurised and fast-paced hospital or clinical setting, where timeliness and accuracy are of paramount importance. Days are carefully scheduled with treatments, tests, and nursing care. 'Slow nursing', which originated in the USA, is more of a slow-moving, 'sit-on-the-bed-and-talk' kind of nursing. It takes time to get to know the patients and their worries, problems and hopes, and to support them. Patients and service users with a learning disability must feel comfortable with the nurse, must be able to trust them before allowing that nurse to work with them. The building up of a culture of mutual trust and confidence is likely to be a vital aspect of spiritual connectedness.

THE ROLE OF THE NURSE

As a nurse, you have a professional responsibility to take into account and accommodate the spiritual beliefs and practices of those with learning disabilities during the provision of care, and to safeguard the right to hold and express such beliefs. This holds true regardless of where you work.

First of all, it is vital that you are aware of, comfortable with and understand your own spiritual identity and journey. Without such awareness and understanding, it may be difficult to engage with the spiritual identity and journey of another (Barber, 2013). Allow the patient or service user to gently guide you and take the lead in their own spiritual dance. Always give those with a learning disability space to share – and care professionals the space to listen (Swinton, 2001). It may be helpful to compile a calendar of major spiritual and religious festivals and understand the spiritual significance of these festivals in the lives of people.

Those with severe or profound and multiple learning disabilities may experience major communication difficulties. This can lead to difficulties in expressing beliefs or participating in activities that are considered part of the life of a particular faith community. Therefore, take time to really communicate and listen to your patients and service users.

Some belief systems attach particular importance to personal hygiene before prayer, with hygiene being intimately linked to concepts of inner cleanliness and purity. Those who possess such beliefs and have a learning disability may need more regular assistance with washing whilst on the ward or in the care home.

At all times, privacy is to be maintained. As well as being understood in terms of the right to privacy, access to personal space and time alone is an important aspect of allowing individuals to develop their understanding of their world, reflect on their circumstances and beliefs, pray or otherwise contemplate their environment and how they relate to it.

It is vital for the nurse to be aware of and forge links/bridges with resources such as local faith communities that could be of use to those with a learning disability (Gaventa, 2010). Such links may prove useful in encouraging faith community leaders to engage with patients and service users who have a learning disability whilst they are in your care. Nurses who work specifically with those who have a learning disability will also have a role in facilitating and participating in the training of both nursing and medical colleagues and local faith communities and their leaders. Such participation in the training of nursing and medical colleagues and faith communities could include presenting at team meetings, running or being involved in workshops or seminars aimed at nurses or faith community leaders or presenting at conferences. It may also be useful to submit posters to various conferences that are targeted at health care assistants and allied care professionals.

CONCLUSION

Whilst great care must be taken not to impose one's own personal beliefs (because to do so can be seen as abusive), spirituality can often be seen as a very personal, complex, fulfilling yet challenging and confusing way of expressing oneself. This is even more so when people have a learning disability, as a result of the differing ways in which they communicate, engage and interact with the world, the environment and the people around them. It is as unethical and unprofessional to ignore, downplay, patronise or belittle the importance of spirituality in the lives of those with a learning disability, as it is to engage with and treat anyone else in like manner.

> **KEY POINTS**
>
> ☞ Those with a learning disability have as much right and need to express their spirituality as anyone else.
>
> ☞ Spirituality has a number of meanings, with many of these meanings involving a personal search for meaning and purpose in life which may or may not be related to religion.
>
> ☞ Many of those with a learning disability are likely to experience a number of barriers to a personal expression of an authentic spirituality.
>
> ☞ There are a number of resources that can be of use to those with a learning disability, to nurses or to both.
>
> ☞ The role of the nurse is to be aware of and understand the importance of spirituality in people's lives and to act appropriately on this awareness and understanding.

REFERENCES

Barber, C. (2013) Article 6: spirituality and learning disability. *British Journal of Health Care Assistants*, 7:4; 180–185.

Faith and Light Communities (2012) www.faithandlight.org.uk (last accessed 16 October 2014)

Gaventa, W. (2010) Spirituality issues and strategies. *In* Friedman, S. & Helm, D. (2010) *End-of-life Care for Children and Adults with Intellectual and Developmental Disabilities.* American Association on Intellectual and Developmental Disabilities, Washington, DC.

L'Arche (2013) www.larche.org.uk (last accessed 16 October 2014)

MacKinlay, E. (2006) *Spiritual growth and care in the fourth age of life.* London, Jessica Kingsley Publishers.

Males, J. & Boswell, C. (1990) Spiritual needs of people with a mental handicap. *Nursing Standard,* 4(48): 35–7.

McSherry, W. (2007) *The Meaning of Spirituality and Spiritual Care within Nursing and Health Care Practice.* London, Quay Books.

Murray, R. & Zentner, J. (1989) *Nursing Concepts for Health Promotion.* London, Prentice Hall.

Reed, P. (1992) An emerging paradigm for the investigation of spirituality in nursing. *Research in Nursing and Health,* 15: 349–57.

Schneiders, S. (1989) Spirituality in the academy. *Theological Studies,* 50: 678–97.

Stoll, R. (1989) The essence of spirituality. *In* Carson, V. (1989) *Spiritual Dimensions of Nursing Practice.* Philadelphia, W.B. Saunders.

Swinton, J. (2001) *A Space to Listen: meeting the spiritual needs of people with learning disabilities.* Foundation for People with Learning Disabilities, London.

Swinton, J. (2002) Spirituality and the lives of people with learning disabilities: a review. *Tizard Learning Disability Review,* 7(4): 29–35.

Tanyi, R. (2002) Towards clarification of the meaning of spirituality. *Journal of Advanced Nursing,* 39(5): 500–509.

The Kairos Forum (2013) www.thekairosforum.com/ (last accessed 16 October 2014)

Wiseman, J. (2006) *Spirituality and Mysticism.* Orbis Books.

15

THE FUTURE AND LEARNING DISABILITY

AIMS AND LEARNING OUTCOMES:

The aims of this chapter are to:

- Summarise a number of the key points that have been made throughout this book

- Highlight the current situation with regard to support and care for those with a learning disability

- Highlight a number of possible future issues regarding such support and care.

By the end of this chapter, the nurse will be:

- Reminded of many of the issues highlighted in previous chapters

- Able to discuss the position of those with a learning disability and learning disability with regard to care and support

- Able to discuss possible future issues regarding those with a learning disability and their care and support.

INTRODUCTION

Sally: As the seven of us were mentioned in the opening chapter to this book, I thought it would be fitting to conclude this book with us. You are all very welcome to my home; please help yourselves to the tea, coffee and cakes.

Chris: Although Thomas has a profound and multiple learning disability (PMLD) and would thus not normally be able to communicate verbally, for the purpose and duration of this chapter he needs to do so and I am exercising 'author's privilege', meaning that Thomas is now able to talk so as to contribute his views and ideas to this conversation, even though this may be seen as 'cheating'. I hope that you don't mind. Again, I am here as the 'author' of this book although I have been rather silent in terms of the care scenarios and dialogues that have occurred in previous chapters.

Hanif: Thanks Chris. I thought that it may be useful to revisit some of the key points that have been raised throughout this book.

Ziva: It may also be useful to briefly discuss our present before discussing our future. As I have Asperger's, I include myself in this 'our'. How's this for an opening thought: "If the people that are brought together by this label of learning disability share one thing in common, it is the potential to be marginalised within the health care system (Griffiths *et al.*, 2008)".

THE PAST: A SUMMARY

Marcel: I think that the definitions and meanings of learning disability that Chris outlined in *Chapter 2* were fair, accurate and OK. Do you agree, Thomas?

Thomas: Yes, particularly when he outlined and briefly discussed a number of these definitions. I particularly agree with Chris's assertion that unless one is able to understand what learning disability is, it could be suggested that health and social care and support of those with a learning disability will be impoverished.

Sally: That's a bit heavy, isn't it? After all, I don't need to understand cancer to provide good quality nursing care to those with cancer…

Thomas: Maybe not. However, if you want to provide more than basic, although good quality, nursing care it would help if you did know enough about cancer to provide that care. Surely, the same applies to providing good quality nursing care to myself, Marcel, Jill's sister, Ziva and other people who have a learning disability or autism spectrum conditions.

Sally: Point taken. This is particularly important when providing nursing care and support to those with profound and multiple learning disabilities such as yourself, Thomas. This may sound strange but as a general / adult nurse, I am more at home with addressing the physical manifestations and meeting the needs of profound disability such as mobility issues, pain management, personal hygiene and dressing, eating, drinking, elimination and breathing.

Jill: In all fairness, Thomas and Marcel, this is perhaps right and proper although I agree that as general nurses we should perhaps be more aware of and understand the whole person behind all these physical health issues.

Hanif: What did you think about *Chapter 4* on legislation? Was there anything that Chris left out?

Ziva: I think that, given the complexity of legislation and the various government and independent reports around learning disability services and care over the past 40-odd years, that it was fair and accurate as far as it went. Perhaps there is a need for a greater discussion around certain pieces of law and their impact upon those with a learning disability, particularly in relation to discrimination, and the 'Family and Children's Bill' that is currently going through parliament was missed out. This could perhaps form the basis of an additional chapter in any updated version of this book.

Chris: Sorry about that and point taken.

Marcel: Your fifth chapter, that of caring for myself and Thomas within a general hospital setting perhaps forms the centre of your book as possibly most of those who will buy and read it are likely to be working within an acute general hospital. Would you say that is fair, Chris?

Chris: Yes, and again either a much longer chapter or perhaps two, three or four chapters or even a whole book that focuses on providing good quality nursing care in these settings would have been helpful. Perhaps a much slimmer book that focused purely on nursing care in these settings may be called for.

Thomas: Chris, I notice that you have not included a chapter on the history of learning disability. Why was this?

Chris: Tony Gilbert (Gilbert, 2009) has already done this and to some depth; I did not see the point of repeating him. Having said that, I believe that it is vital to have a basic understanding of the history of learning disability and learning disability care; without such understanding we are condemned to repeat its mistakes.

Marcel: Thank you Chris for including chapters on sexuality, old age, death and spirituality. These are important although very difficult issues to get to grips with. Having said that, these issues are likely to have profound effects on all of us – sexuality and spirituality have such a major impact on our identity as human beings and yet strangely tend to be forgotten by other writers. Such omissions by other people tend to make our lives poorer.

Ziva: Chris, I read *Chapter 12* on care givers with great interest and could not help but notice the anger that was expressed. Good! It would have been only too easy to have let nursing and medical staff off the hook by claiming that care givers do not experience significant difficulties in their caring responsibilities at the hands of care professionals.

Chris: Thanks, Ziva. I agree there was a lot of frustration and pain rather than anger and I stand by my decision not to 'airbrush' this frustration and pain out of the text. To have done so neither respects care givers nor is likely to bring about change. Likewise with *Chapter 13* on disability discrimination; no-one is served well by trying to deny that disability discrimination exists and can have a profound effect on both individuals and society.

THE PRESENT

Sally: So, where are we now?

Marcel: Apart from sitting in your lounge and eating your cakes you mean? Well, I think that most health and social care services are gradually getting there. Hospitals, GP practices and community health centres know that we exist and are beginning to understand that our health needs, that my health needs are both the same as and different from yours. We are being treated more as individuals and less as a large group. However, there is still the idea that a 'one size fits all' approach exists, lurking behind the scenes.

Thomas: I agree with you, Marcel. On the plus side, there appears to be greater awareness, understanding and appreciation on the part of health and social care professionals regarding the existence and needs of you and me and others who have a learning disability. This has resulted in a much improved nursing practice and hence the services that we experience. And please never forget that this is as much about the services that we *experience* as it is about services that are *delivered*. However, on the minus side there is still much that needs to be done.

Chris: What do you mean, Thomas? Surely, services that are delivered are the same as the services that are experienced?

Thomas: Not necessarily, Chris. Yes, in an ideal world it would be. However, whilst you as a care professional may wholeheartedly believe that you are giving of your best, I as a patient or service user may perceive and experience a crap service!

Marcel: Well said, Thomas. In a nutshell, this could be a somewhat crude soundbite summary of the 2007 Mencap report '*Death by Indifference*'! And don't forget that Mencap has produced a number of follow-up reports since this initial 2007 report, all of which have suggested that, far from improving, nurses' knowledge about, attitudes towards and care for those with learning disabilities have not improved. We haven't even got around to mentioning, let alone discussing, Winterbourne View yet or the fallout from Mid-Stafford hospital... and that poor quality care for those with a learning disability is likely to have been endemic in such environments.

THE FUTURE

Ziva: I can hear the anger in your voices, Marcel and Thomas, and as a person who is on the autism spectrum I can really understand how you feel. Can I ask you all four questions: where do you see, and where would you like to see those with a learning disability in, say, twenty years' time? Where do you see, and where would you like to see learning disability services in twenty years' time? As you wrote this book, Chris, can I ask you to start?

Chris: Thanks Ziva! Well, I think that we will be looking more at a far greater understanding of those with a learning disability and their needs on the part of the non-learning disability specialist, an understanding that is matched by perhaps a slower and more gradual evolution rather than revolution in terms of changes in service delivery. That is not to say that changes in awareness, understanding and service delivery will not happen, as clearly they will and I hope that this small book would have played a tiny part in that change. I think that Marcel,

Jill's sister and Thomas – Marcel in particular – will be more involved in the teaching and training of health and social care staff through presenting at conferences, teaching nursing students or running workshops. I would like to see Marcel and Thomas more in control of how and where they live, what they do, their finances and how and where they spend their money. Any thoughts, Marcel?

Marcel: I like the idea of being in control of my own destiny. However, I am also aware that there are institutions like Winterbourne View out there and I don't believe for one moment that this was a single rogue institution. Bad practices will continue to exist and possibly flourish in such institutions and those like me and my friends will continue to be both accidentally and even deliberately harmed within their walls whilst the world turns its back on us.

Chris: That's a sad thing to say, Marcel! Surely, the whole point of this book is to contribute to the improving of awareness and understanding amongst 'non-specialist' health care professionals?

Marcel: Yes, Chris, it probably will do and thanks also for allowing Thomas and me to share our stories, our hopes, our thoughts and our lives within these pages. It is greatly appreciated. However, as long as there are people such as Collin Brewer and Nick Martin, the local politicians who were briefly mentioned in *Chapter 13* on disability discrimination, there will also be people and institutions that will treat us as trash!

Sally: Hang on a minute. Who are Collin Brewer and Nick Martin?

Marcel: Sorry for mentioning these people again as they have already been mentioned during a previous discussion in *Chapter 13*. However, I believe that it is important to mention these people again. Brewer was a local politician in Cornwall (Mencap, 2013) who stated that children with a disability are like deformed lambs and should be killed in the same way that farmers would put down a disabled or sick animal. He believed that the money that would be saved through the killing of disabled children would open and run ten public toilets. He also appears to be unrepentant about his comments. Nick Martin was the mayor of Swindon until April 2014 who asked whether 'mongols' such as me and Jill's sister were still allowed to have sex. I also don't believe that Brewer and Martin were and are the only people to hold such extreme views. So if you put Brewer and Martin together with Winterbourne View, you end up with a very poisonous mix indeed!

Sally: Thanks for that Marcel. As a senior staff nurse working in an acute medical ward, I would like to see future care services for those with a learning disability being provided on grounds of quality rather than cost. However, given the very tight funding of health care services, I feel that cost rather than quality will dictate health care service provision.

Chris: I agree and it is up to all of us to ensure that those with a learning disability don't lose out as a result! We need to generate a culture of 'bottom up' change rather than 'top down' dictates.

Sally: I would also like to see those with a learning disability being used or employed as 'lay assessors', as 'mystery shoppers' to assess all aspects of health care support and services with their feedback being heard, listened to, understood and acted upon. Partnership working between people with a learning disability and service providers at all levels of health care organisations (from health care assistants and student nurses to nurse directors) would also be really interesting and useful, with all partners being of equal level.

Thomas: The problem here is, would the relatively powerful nurse directors welcome the idea of treating Marcel and me as equals? If not, then what would be the point? If we are not treated as equals then it is just lip service, window dressing. I'm not into window dressing! Having said that, there are in many areas of the UK learning disability, autism and mental health partnership boards which do have quite powerful self-advocacy input. These partnership boards come into their own when feeding into and implementing local, regional and national initiatives, strategies and services. However, for these boards to work well it needs to be genuine partnership rather than window dressing.

Hanif: I would like to see a national service framework (NSF) for those with learning disabilities that sets out both the general and more specific directions for service commissioning and delivery at national, regional and local levels. At the moment, learning disability is one of the conditions that does not have such a framework although the NSF for 'long-term conditions' is perhaps the 'best fit' in terms of appropriateness. This could perhaps be followed by a law that focuses specifically on learning disability, particularly in adults, in much the same way as the Autism Act 2009 did for adults on the autism spectrum. At the moment, the Autism Act is the only disability-specific law that we have. I would also see many of those with a learning disability self-advocating in terms of being actively involved in contributing to both any NSFs and legislation. However, this may involve a massive redistribution of power from existing politicians, service designers and commissioners.

Ziva: The question is: are those who hold and exercise such relative power willing or likely to really share that power? I'm not entirely sure that they will ever be! To change the subject a bit, I would like to see a much greater interdisciplinary and multi-professional training at both under- and postgraduate levels. Such interdisciplinary training and networking is already happening but it needs to improve. I would also like to see Marcel, Thomas and Jill's sister being heavily involved in facilitating and leading such training and networks. I would hope that such interdisciplinary training would lead to genuine holistic and multidisciplinary care and support assessments, planning, implementation and evaluation where the person with a learning disability is at the centre rather than the periphery, and is fully involved rather than being a passive recipient of this process. Having said that, I am fully aware of some of the barriers to such holistic working including 'professional politics', professional accountability, management structures and different ways of working. I suppose these could be summed up in the phrase 'different power structures' which brings us back again to the idea of real and genuine power sharing amongst all those involved.

Jill: In my experience, as 'mainstream' NHS services and their general trained nursing staff appear to be 'ill-equipped' to support those such as my sister, who has Down's syndrome, who need to access generic hospital services, I believe that there is a need for specialist nursing support. I know that there are learning disability liaison nurses in many acute hospitals; but is that enough? Just a thought! I also believe that commissioners and senior managers of clinical services must have a clinical background and such background should be fairly recent; it should also include working with those who have a learning disability. I believe that without such a background, service commissioners would not have a clue about how to support those with a learning disability.

Ziva: Just another thought, as those with a learning disability and those who are on the autism spectrum such as me and you, Chris, could be seen as simply a 'variant of the human condition'; do we need specialist health care services, nursing or otherwise? After all, such services can be quite expensive and in a very 'cash-strapped' health care environment...

Marcel: I fear, in that case, that we will return to the old institutions where choice, dignity and respect did not exist. Those who lived in these old hospitals still tell me of bath times when three service users were being bathed at the same time and in the same bath room: one getting undressed, one being bathed and one getting dried and dressed again. It would mean going back to a time when everyone got hot tea which was served in huge metal tea pots with milk and loads of sugar already added, whether people liked tea or not, whether they liked sugar with their tea or not. There was no choice.

Thomas: I think that all of us, those with a learning disability and nurses, need to be much more proactive in ensuring that largely historical events and people don't exist in the future.

Chris: Sorry for interrupting but I am assuming here that these events and people refer to Winterbourne View, Mencap reports into deaths due to poor nursing care and people like Collin Brewer and Nick Martin (see *Chapter 13* for a fuller explanation of these)? I agree that whilst these are historical in nature, they have a huge impact upon the future. I also agree that it is up to all of us to ensure that these historical events and people stay where they belong, in the past.

Thomas: You are right, Chris. I think that it is fitting that Marcel and I should have the last words here. I think that we all agree that the future of both those with a learning disability and learning disability services isn't looking too bad and that those with a learning disability such as us could and perhaps are likely to have a significant impact upon staff training and development and deciding what and how health care support services are planned, delivered and implemented.

Marcel: Finally, major changes in learning disability services have usually been driven by ideology and money. However, please do not confuse change with progress! People have very good intentions; most people are saying the right things. But without the political will and the money that goes with it, nothing will change and in twenty years' time we could still have Winterbournes, Collin Brewers, Nick Martins and Mencap reports into poor nursing and medical care.

REFERENCES

Gilbert, T. (2009) From the workhouse to citizenship: four ages of learning disability. *In* Jukes, M. (2009) *Learning Disability Nursing Practice*. London, Quay Books.

Griffiths, P., Winterhalder, R., Clark, L. & Hicks, A. (2008) The future of services for intellectual impairment. *In* Clark, L. & Griffiths, P. (2008) *Learning Disability and Other Intellectual Impairments: meeting needs through health services*. Chichester, Wiley.

Mencap (2013) *Mencap calls for the resignation of Collin Brewer*. Available at: www.mencap. org.uk/news/article/mencap-calls-resignation-collin-brewer-0

GLOSSARY

AS: Asperger's syndrome; the 'higher IQ' end of the autism spectrum.

ASC: Autism spectrum condition, ranging from 'classic autism' through to Asperger's syndrome. There are about 670 000 people in the UK (about 1.1% of the UK population) who are on the autism spectrum.

ASD: Autism spectrum disorder. ASD and ASC are often used interchangeably. Some people prefer the term 'condition' whilst others use 'disorder'.

AS/HFA: Asperger's syndrome / high-functioning autism.

Developmental delay: The term that is currently used in the USA to designate those with a learning disability. This has largely taken over from the term 'mental retardation' (The American Association on Mental Retardation continued to use the term *mental retardation* until 2006).

Down's syndrome: Down's syndrome is a genetic condition caused by the presence of an extra chromosome in the body's cells. Down's syndrome is not a disease, and it is not a hereditary condition. It occurs by chance at conception. Everyone with Down's syndrome will have some degree of learning disability. Certain physical characteristics and health conditions are common among people with Down's syndrome. Down's syndrome used to be called 'mongolism'.

Epilepsy: Epilepsy is a neurological condition which affects around 600 000 people in the UK (1% of the UK population) where there is a tendency to experience recurrent seizures (fits), of which there are around 40 different types. Epilepsy can affect anyone, from any walk of life and from any age. For more information see: www.epilepsy.org.uk/press/facts.

Learning disability:
- An arrested or incomplete development of mind
- A significantly reduced ability to understand new or complex information (impaired intelligence and cognitive functioning)

- A significantly reduced ability to learn new skills (impaired intelligence and cognitive functioning), with
- A reduced ability to cope independently (impaired social functioning) and
- Which started before adulthood and with a lasting effect on development.

Mencap: A voluntary sector organisation that raises the profile of, and campaigns for those with a learning disability and their families. Their services are UK-wide.

Mental handicap: An older term used to designate those with a learning disability that was used throughout the 1980s and early 1990s.

Mental retardation: An older term used to designate those with a learning disability that was used throughout the 1960s.

Mental subnormality: An older term used to designate those with a learning disability that was used throughout the 1970s.

Nurse: A nurse is a person who has successfully undergone three years of training and preparation, usually at undergraduate / first degree level, and is registered with and regulated by the Nursing and Midwifery Council (NMC). Other countries are likely to have similar training and registration requirements. This is distinct from health or social care assistants or nursing assistants / auxiliaries who do not embark upon or complete nurse training and, at the moment, are not professionally registered and regulated.

RN(LD): Registered nurse (learning disability): the current learning disability nurse qualification and NMC entry.

RN(MH): Registered nurse (mental handicap): an older learning disability nurse qualification used throughout the 1980s.

RN(MS): Registered nurse (mental subnormality): an older learning disability nurse qualification used throughout the 1970s.

RESOURCES

BILD: British Institute of Learning Disability. BILD uses its books and journals, conferences and events, and membership information and networks to encourage the exchange of new ideas and good practice. BILD also provides consultancy and, through support for the health and social care qualifications and training in the workplace, can help support the development of staff and the organisations they work for. BILD can be contacted at:
BILD, Birmingham Research Park, 97 Vincent Drive, Edgbaston, Birmingham B15 2SQ.
By telephone: 0121 415 6960; by fax: 0121 415 6999
By email: enquiries@bild.org.uk

Carers UK: One of the two main voluntary sector organisations specifically for 'informal care givers'. Carers UK provide a wide range of information both for care givers and for care professionals, run care giver support groups throughout the UK and campaign on care giver issues locally, regionally and nationally. Their website is www.carersuk.org

Cerebra: Founded in 2001, Cerebra is a unique national charity that strives to improve the lives of children with brain-related neurological conditions such as learning disability and autism spectrum conditions, through research, education and direct, ongoing support. Their website is: www.cerebra.org.uk/

Down's Syndrome Association: Provides information and support on all aspects of Down's syndrome to all who require it. Their website is: www.downs-syndrome.org.uk/
(Information regarding a number of other forms of learning disability such as Rett syndrome and tuberous sclerosis can also be found on the internet).

Houses of Parliament all-party interest group on learning disability: This is a group of MPs and peers who have a special interest in learning disability issues. Its internet address is www.publications.parliament.uk/pa/cm/cmallparty/register/learning-disability.htm

Kairos: Kairos was established by John Swinton (professor of practical theology at the University of Aberdeen) and Christina Gangemi to provide advice, information, advocacy, and support for individuals who have a learning disability and their families regarding spirituality, religious practice and the vital role they have within communities. The creation of a space for the development of networks of lay people, professionals and religious communities was seen as crucial as a way of providing information regarding spirituality and learning disability (www.thekairosforum.com/).

KIDS: KIDS is a UK voluntary sector organisation which, in its 40-year history, has pioneered a number of approaches and programmes for children and young people who have a disability. These include home learning (Portage), parent partnerships, adventure playgrounds and the inclusion of children with disabilities in mainstream settings. Its website is: www.kids.org.uk/

L'Arche: In a world that places such value on success and winning, L'Arche communities are places where people can take time to explore who they are, not just what they can do. They are places of welcome where people are transformed by an intense experience of community, relationship, disability and difference. Set up by Jean Vanier, L'Arche is an international voluntary sector organisation that provides residential services for those with a learning disability along broadly Christian lines. Its website is www.larche.org.uk/

Learning disability liaison nurses: Learning disability liaison nurses are specialist learning disability nurses who are increasingly based in general/acute hospitals. Their main roles include:
- Working in collaboration with the acute hospital to enable open and easy access to health care services for people with learning disabilities
- Being a point of contact and resource for the non-learning disability specialist
- Working at a strategic level with health professionals, managers and commissioners to achieve the health agenda of the White Paper *Valuing People*.

They can be contacted via the hospital switchboard.

Learning Disability Practice: A monthly peer-reviewed journal from the publishing arm of the Royal College of Nursing (RCN Publishing); it can be viewed on their website: http://learningdisabilitypractice.rcnpublishing.co.uk/

Learning Disabilities Public Health Observatory, Lancaster University: The Health Observatory is an aspect of the Centre for Disability Research and is headed by Professor Eric Emerson. The Improving Health and Lives Learning Disabilities Observatory exists to monitor the health of people with learning disabilities and the health care they receive. Their website is www.improvinghealthandlives.org.uk/

Mencap: Mencap is one of the main voluntary sector organisations that campaigns for those with a learning disability and provides support, information and advocacy for those with a learning disability, their families and care professionals nationally, regionally and locally. Their website is www.mencap.org.uk/

Mind: Mind is one of a wide range of voluntary sector organisations that provide information, support and campaign for those who experience mental health issues, their families and care professionals. Their website is www.mind.org.uk/

Naidex: Naidex National is the home of the UK independent living market. It is the largest UK exhibition and conference of its kind, showcasing a comprehensive range of products, services and workshops/seminars that enable people with a disability to live more independently. Naidex takes place each April or May at the NEC, Birmingham. The Naidex website is: www.naidex.co.uk/

National Autistic Society (NAS): One of the main organisations that raises the profile of and campaigns for those on the autism spectrum and provides information about autism spectrum conditions for those on the spectrum, their families and care professionals. Their council and trustee board includes those who are on the autism spectrum. Their website is: www.nas.org.uk

Princess Royal Trust for Carers: One of the two main voluntary sector organisations specifically for 'informal care givers'. The Princess Royal Trust for Carers campaigns and offers advice, information and support for informal carers and care professionals. Its website is www.carers.org/

Reports on learning disability care: There have been a large number of official reports into the care of those with a learning disability over the past 40 years. See *Chapter 4* for a list of these.

Scope: Scope is a national voluntary sector organisation that raises the profile of people with disabilities through providing information, campaigning and offering a range of services for children and adults with disabilities; it is primarily focused on those with complex support needs. Its website is www.scope.org.uk/

Support groups: There are a wide variety of support groups for those with a learning disability, their parents and their siblings. At the moment, whether there are any support groups specifically for children of those with a learning disability is unknown. In the first instance, contact your local or regional Mencap branch/office or the hospital's learning disability liaison nurse for advice and possible contact details.

UK legislation: Information regarding a wide range of UK laws/legislation, Parliamentary Bills, White Papers and related issues can be found at the UK Government's website: www.legislation.gov.uk/
Examples of such legislation would include:
- The Mental Capacity Act 2005: www.legislation.gov.uk/ukpga/2005/9/contents
- The Autism Act 2009: www.legislation.gov.uk/ukpga/2009/15/contents
- The Equality Act 2010: www.legislation.gov.uk/ukpga/2010/15/contents

INDEX

If you wish to follow the views/thoughts of the individuals who appear in this book, their names are in speech marks in the index